The Internet for Nurses and Allied Health Professionals

Third Edition

Springer

New York
Berlin
Heidelberg
Barcelona
Hong Kong
London
Milan
Paris
Singapore
Tokyo

THE
INTERNET
FOR
NURSES
AND ALLIED HEALTH PROFESSIONALS

THIRD EDITION

with 29 Illustrations

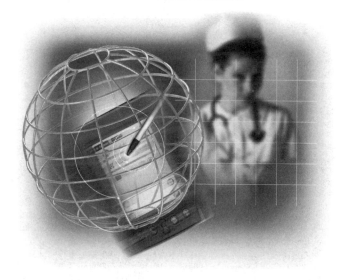

MARGARET J.A. EDWARDS

Margaret J.A. Edwards & Associates, Inc.
Calgary, Alberta
Canada

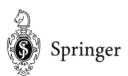 Springer

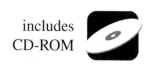 includes
CD-ROM

Margaret J.A. Edwards
Margaret J.A. Edwards & Associates, Inc.
52 Canova Road SW
Calgary, AB T2W 2A6
Canada

Library of Congress Cataloging-in-Publication Data
Edwards, Margaret J.A.
    The Internet for nurses and allied health professionals / Margaret J.A. Edwards.—3rd ed.
    p. ; cm.
    Includes bibliographical references and index.
    ISBN 0-387-95236-5 (s/c : alk. paper)
    1. Nursing—Computer network resources.   2. Internet.   3. Medical care—Computer
network resources.   4. Allied health personnel.   I. Title.
    [DNLM: 1. Computer Communications Networks—Nurses' Instruction.   2. Allied Health
Personnel—Nurses' Instruction.   3. Information Systems—Nurses' Instruction. WY 26.5
E26i 2001]
RT50.5 .E36 2001
004.67′8′—dc21   2001031417

Printed on acid-free paper.

Production managed by A. Orrantia; manufacturing supervised by Jerome Basma.
Typeset by Robert Wexler, Yellow Springs, OH.
Printed and bound by R.R. Donnelley and Sons, Harrisonburg, PA.
Printed in the United States of America.

9 8 7 6 5 4 3 2 1

ISBN 0-387-95236-5   SPIN 10792837

Springer-Verlag   New York Berlin Heidelberg
A member of BertelsmannSpringer Science+Business Media GmbH

Preface

The INTERNET. Everyone is talking about it. The newspapers report new applications daily. Even the kids at school are connected! But does the Internet offer anything beyond endless shopping at cybermalls, a plethora of computer games or a worldwide club for computer nerds? Is there anything out there for nurses and allied health professionals? YES, there is! That's what this book is all about.

This book is designed as a primer to the Internet for nurses and allied health professionals who have little or no computer experience. In plain language we will describe the Internet and how it works. We'll outline the ways in which the Internet can be a valuable partner in your practice. Information about using various Internet tools will be given. Finally, we've done some of the searching for you and will provide a catalogue of Internet resources that we found, with access directions and a brief summary of each resource. We have not attempted to make this catalogue a massive "yellow pages" directory to all health-related sites. Rather, we have identified key sites related to each topic. Sites included are good starting places for searches and generally include links to other Internet resources.

If, in addition to being a health professional, you are a "techie," who is already well-grounded in the fundamentals of the Internet, you will probably find the chapters to be mostly review. However, you'll find the compilation of health-related resources in the catalogue to be valuable.

Health care is changing daily. Nurses and allied health professionals are scrambling to keep up with an ever-changing "healthscape". Traditional methods of formally communicating with peers through conferences, journals and books are not able to provide the answers that health care providers require in a timely manner. When you need to know now how others have dealt with a proposed health care change, you can't wait three months for the next conference or nine months for the book to come out. This is where you discover the real power of the Internet. Your ability to immediately ask questions or exchange ideas with peers around the world gives you the knowledge edge you need to keep your nursing or health care practice professional and progressive.

The INTERNET... How did we ever manage without it!

Contents

Acknowledgments

The preparation and production of any book requires the input of many people. Nhora Cortes-Comerer, Michelle Schmitt and Tony Orrantia at Springer-Verlag graciously provided both support and technical expertise. Darren Bierman produced the line art.

I would like to acknowledge the enormous contribution of my husband, Craig Edwards, in supporting the preparation of the manuscript and preparing the copy. Special thanks to my mother, Mary Burchell, and sister, Rosemary Burchell, for child-care above and beyond the call of duty! Finally, my thanks to my children for eating a lot of pizza and giving up the computer (and their mother) while the book was prepared. Thank you all!

M.J.A.E.

Part One
Introduction

Part One
Introduction

1
Internet Basics

What is the Internet?

At the most basic level, the Internet is the name for a group of worldwide computer-based information resources connected together. It is often defined as a network of networks of computers. Today, according to the Internet Society, there are more than 93 million hosts (computers) connected throughout the world. These hosts support over 1 billion indexable Web pages. Every week, it is estimated that over 1 million sites join the Internet.

One of the major challenges in using the Internet is that there is no clear map of how all those networks are connected. There is also no master list of what information or resource is available where! Because there is no overall structured grand plan, the shape and face of the Internet are constantly changing to meet the needs of the people who use it. The Internet can be likened to a cloud in this way; it's amorphous, without boundaries and constantly changing shape and space. Even in the catalogue that we offer in this book, there are entries whose location has changed from the time we write about them to the time you try to find them according to our instructions.

Although the thought of all those computers joined together is mind-boggling, the real power of the Internet is in the people and information that all those computers connect. The Internet is really a people-oriented community that allows millions of people around the world to communicate with one another. Amazingly, people voluntarily share their time, ideas, and products, for the most part without any personal or financial gain. The computers move the information around and execute the programs that allow us to access the information. However, it is the information itself and the people connected to the information that make the Internet useful and recreational!

Who Owns and Operates the Internet?

The statistics on the massive size and astronomical growth of the Internet would lead us to believe that somewhere there is a super-organization holding it all together. The reality of the Internet organization is very different. The Internet is not "owned" by anyone, in the usual sense of the word. The organizations and individuals that use the Internet manage and pay for their own pieces through a system that looks a lot like anarchy! There are no CEOs or corporate boards of directors, but rather the Internet is "governed" by a loose confederation of users.

Each organization or individual pays for its own computers and networks and co-operates with its neighbor networks to pay for the communication lines that connect them. Regional networks are an example of this type of organization. In my city, several university departments, four major hospitals, and eight community and private sector organizations, each maintaining their own computer systems, have worked together to develop a network connection between them all. This network is called "Agenet." It is used to send information about aging among the local network members. The expense of developing and maintaining this local network is the responsibility of the members. Grants, tax money, dues, and university and corporate monies are funding sources for these local networks. This example is played out millions of times around the world. Leased lines can then connect local networks to each other. Consortiums of local networks and organizations then pool their purchasing power to obtain leased lines and better support for their members. In this way, you can see that it is the often unstated cooperation of organizations and individuals that allows the Internet to function without specific management. The Internet, then, is owned by nobody and everybody.

In many countries, the "backbone" of the Internet in that country is funded by government organizations. In the United States, the National Science Foundation (NSF) originally funded the backbone. Supercomputer centers were established around the United States by the National Science Foundation in the mid-1980s. To provide universities and research centers around the country with remote access to these supercomputers, the National Science Foundation funded a backbone network (NSFNET) that connected these supercomputer centers. NSF also provided the funding for connections to the backbone for regional networks. In 1995, due to the growth in commercial network providers, NSFNET reverted to a research network. The main backbone traffic in the United States is now routed through those interconnected commercial network providers. In Canada, CA*net Networking Inc. was formed in 1990 to manage the Internet backbone for Canada, appropriately called CA*net. CA*net is run by a group called CANARIE (Canadian Network for the Advancement of Research, Industry and Education). In 1998, Canada launched CA*net 3, the first national optical Internet backbone.

Although there is no specific governance of the Internet, voluntary co-ordinating and overseeing of the workings of the networks is done by the Internet Society. The Internet Society fosters the continued evolution of the Internet through education, support for technical development, and provision of a forum for exploring new Internet applications. Membership in this nonprofit society is open to any organization or individual. Additionally, any network connected to the Internet agrees to the decisions and standards established by the

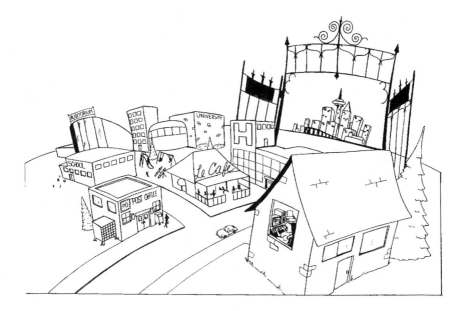

Figure 1.1 An Electronic Town.

Internet Architecture Board (IAB). Anyone willing to help can participate in the process of setting standards.

What Does the Internet Look Like?

We want to use two analogies that are particularly graphic in describing the Internet: "the electronic town/global village" and "the Information Highway." Figure 1.1 is a graphic representation of an electronic town.

To begin to understand the electronic town, let's start with small town "FreeNets" before we move on to investigate a large metropolis, "the Internet." A FreeNet is a computer network that brings together the resources of a community or a campus. Just like most small towns, a FreeNet has a post office where members have mailboxes and can send or receive mail from around the world (electronic mail, called e-mail). There is a town square with small restaurants for one-to-one conversations, and auditoriums or a speaker's corner for large gatherings (places on the network called newsgroups or forums). There's also a gateway that enables users to enter other networks around the world. Other organizations on the network are organizations that exist in the real community: schools and universities, hospitals, newsrooms, weather stations, and libraries. All of them are just a telephone call away using your modem and computer! FreeNets exist in most major cities. The biggest problem with FreeNets is the same problem found in many small towns: there are not enough buses in and out of town! In our city of over 750,000 people, there are only 44 connection lines to the FreeNet. That means a lot of standing in line waiting for the bus! We'll talk about ways other than FreeNets to access the Internet in Chapter 2.

If you've driven around small towns, you will have noticed that they all have some unique claim to fame: an airplane museum, the world's most accurate clock, a database of articles on the mating habits of mosquitoes, or the world's biggest supercomputer. Imagine the planet covered with those unique little towns and you have a good picture of the Global Village. Rather than having to drive from one town to another, you can travel to any of these towns with your computer via the Information Highway, the Internet, without ever leaving home. You can look at the Monet collection in the Louvre in Paris with as much ease as using the FreeNet to check local library listings.

Where Did the Internet Come From?

The need to transfer information between computers was recognized soon after computers were developed. At first, this type of information transfer was done by putting the information from one computer onto magnetic tapes or punch cards (remember, this is in the early 1960s). Then you would carry them to another computer where the information could be loaded from the tapes or cards. We still do this today but with files written in ASCII format on a diskette. (This type of a network is called "sneaker net"!). In the 1960s, computer scientists began exploring ways to directly connect remote computers and their users.

In 1969 the United States Department of Defense Advanced Research Projects Agency (ARPA), funded an experimental network called ARPANET. The main goals of the ARPANET research were to link together the Department of Defense and military research contractors that included a large number of universities, and to develop a reliable network. The development of a reliable network involved the concept of dynamic rerouting, which is key to understanding Internet communication today (we'll come back to this concept in Chapter 2). Dynamic rerouting, from the military perspective, would allow communications on a network to be rerouted if part of the network was destroyed by an enemy attack.

The military's goal of a "reliable" network has been accomplished. There are many reports of the Internet being used in "war." Chinese students used their university Internet connections to keep in touch with the world during the Tiananmen Square uprising. Moscow residents used the Internet to report on events during the attempted overthrow of the government in the Soviet Union. Both civilians and the military used Internet routing technology in the Gulf War and the Bosnian conflict.

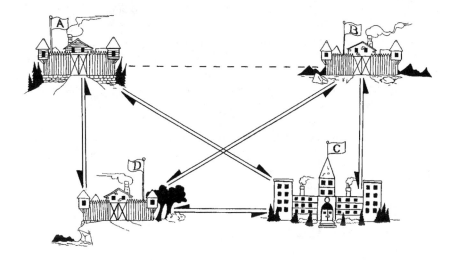

Figure 1.2. Use of Dynamic Rerouting.

Figure 1.2 demonstrates the idea of dynamic rerouting. There are normally direct communication links between all four locations, A, B, C, and D. In Figure 1.2, the direct link between locations A and B has been severed (more likely by a backhoe than an enemy attack!). A and B cannot communicate directly along the dotted line. However, A can still send messages to B in a number of different ways, as indicated by the solid lines in the figure. For example, the message could be routed from A to D and then to B or from A to C and then to B or from A to D to C and then to B. On the Internet, there is always more than one way for the message to move from you to its intended recipient. This is how ARPANET achieved its goal of developing a reliable network.

The ARPANET became very popular and many universities wanted to join it. To accommodate the growing number of sites, the network also had to be able to add and remove new sites easily and to allow computers of many different types to communicate effortlessly. These needs led to the development of the TCP/IP network protocol. TCP/IP (Transmission Control Protocol/Internet Protocol) is the language that computers connected to the ARPANET used to talk to each other. In the early 1980s all the interconnected research networks were converted to the TCP/IP protocol. The ARPANET became the backbone (physical connection) between all the sites. In the mid-1980s the National Science Foundation established supercomputer centers around the United States. The plan for researchers around the United States to use the ARPANET to connect to those supercomputers did not work out, so the National Science Foundation funded the development of NSFNET. In 1990, ARPANET was shut down and NSFNET provided the backbone for Internet communications in the

United States from 1990 to 1995. In 1995, interconnected commercial network providers took over this role in the United States.

In Canada, research networking began in the early 1980s. NetNorth, the Canadian equivalent of the American BitNet organization, was created in early 1984. During the period 1985 to 1988, most of the larger universities began multiyear projects to install high-speed networks on their campuses. Soon, establishing links between these networks and NSFNET became a priority. At the same time, the National Research Council of Canada developed a plan for the creation of a high speed national network. The University of Toronto, in co-operation with IBM Canada and the telecommunications reseller INSINC, won the contract to build this network. In June of 1990, CA*net Networking Inc. was formed to manage the Internet backbone in Canada.

What Is the World Wide Web?

The latest service to be developed in the evolution of attempts to make sense of all the Internet resources is the World Wide Web (variously called WWW, W3, or the Web). The goal of the Web development was to offer a simple, consistent, and intuitive interface to the vast resources of the Internet. The Web tries to provide you with the intuitive links that humans make between information, rather than forcing you to think like a computer and speculate at possible file names and hidden submenus as do the previous services. A short history of the development of the Web will help you understand its services.

History of the Web

In 1989, researchers at CERN (the European Laboratory for Particle Physics) wanted to develop a simpler way of sharing information with a widely dispersed research group. The problems they faced are the same as those you face in using the previous information retrieval systems. Because the researchers were at distant sites, any activity such as reading a shared document or viewing an image required finding the location of the desired information, making a remote connection to the machine containing the information, and then downloading the information to a local machine. Each of these activities required running a variety of applications such as FTP, Telnet, Archie, or an image viewer (see Appendix 2). The researchers decided to develop a system that would allow them to access all types of information from a common interface without the need for all the steps required previously. Between 1990 and 1993, the CERN researchers developed this type of interface, the Web, and the necessary tools to use it. Since 1993, the Web has become the most popular way to access Internet resources.

Hypertext

To navigate around the World Wide Web, you must have a beginning understanding of hypertext. Hypertext is text that contains links to other data. For example, when you are doing a literature search using the hard copy of Cummulative Index of Nursing and Allied Health Literature (CINAHL), you choose your first search term and look it up. As you read through the listings, another idea for a search term comes to you. You put your finger in the first page (so you can return there easily) and turn to the new term. At the bottom of the listings of the second term is a note that says "see also" and gives you several other words to follow. In a hypertext document, you don't have to wait until the end to find the links; they may be anywhere in the document. Links in hypertext documents are marked with color bars, underlining, or square brackets with numbers so that they stand out. Whenever you read a word that is marked as hypertext, you can select it and immediately the link will take you to another document related to the word or phrase. When you have finished looking at the linked document, you simply go back to the previous text, where the program has kept its finger in the page.

This is what makes the Web so powerful. A link may go to any type of Internet resource. For example, the link can take you to a text file, a database of information, a video or audio file, a chat room, or a UseNet newsgroup. Another powerful feature of the Web is that hypertext allows the same piece of information to be linked to hundreds of other documents at the same time. The links can also span traditional boundaries. A hypertext document related to a specific professional group may contain links to information in many different disciplines.

All Web sites have a welcome page, called a home page, that you see when you first connect to that site. The home page may just give the name of the site but usually contains a list of resources and links available at the site. For example, Figure 1.3 is an image of the home page of Springer-Verlag New York (the publisher of this book). If you clicked on the underlined word Medicine on this Web page, the hypertext link would take you to the Web page shown in Figure 1.4. You can continue to select links that will navigate you to the information you are looking for. Or, as we'll discuss in Chapters 7 and 8, you can also use the search engine built into the Springer-Verlag New York Web site to find the information you want more quickly.

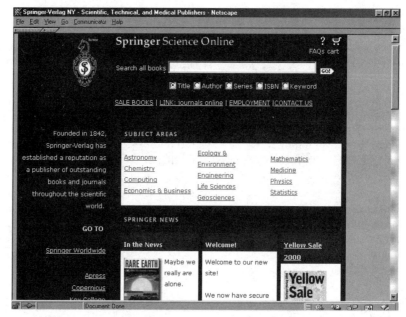

Figure 1.3. The Home Page of Springer-Verlag New York.

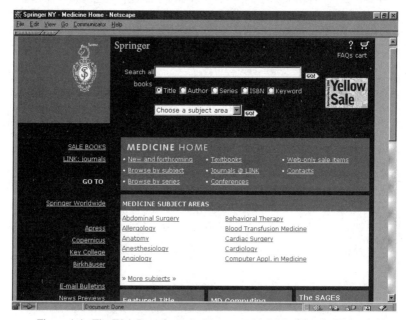

Figure 1.4. The Web Page from the Hypertext Link <u>Medicine</u> in Figure 1.3.

How Do I Get There from Here?

Now that you have an idea of what the Internet is and what the Web can do for you, the next chapter describes various ways of connecting to the Internet and getting you on the Information Highway.

2
Getting Connected

Connecting to the Internet

If you have access to a telephone line, a modem, and a computer, you can connect to the Internet. There are three basic ways to connect to the Internet: make a direct connection over dedicated communications lines, use your computer to connect to a university or hospital computer system that has Internet access, or buy time and connections from a commercial Internet service provider. The next section will describe the various options for connecting to the Internet, including the advantages and disadvantages of each. Then, we'll give some guidelines to help you select the connection that is appropriate for you.

Types of Internet Connections

Direct Connection to the Internet

A direct or dedicated connection wires your computer directly to the Internet through a dedicated machine called a router or gateway. The connection is made over a special kind of telephone line. The gateway makes you an "official" Internet computer that must remain on-line all the time. This type of direct connection is very expensive to install and maintain. For this reason, it is usually used only by large companies or institutions rather than by individuals or small businesses.

Connecting Through Another's Gateway

Another way to connect to the Internet is to use a gateway that another company or institution has established. In this case, a company, university, or hospital that has an Internet gateway allows you to connect to the Internet using its system. The connection is usually made through a modem or remote terminal. This type of access is often available to students through the computing services department of their university. Many hospitals and health services organizations also allow staff access to the Internet through the institution's facilities. This is a good way to begin to learn about the Internet resources that are available, before deciding that you want your own access. The only disadvantage is that the institution may not offer full Internet access, but only e-mail and newsgroup facilities. To use an institution's access, you will need a login ID and password. The information services or computer services department is the place to start inquiring about getting access and authorization to the institution's services. For the individual, this is the best type of access to have if full Internet access is available. Someone other than you maintains the computer system and the Internet connection, and, most importantly, pays for the connection. If you have this type of access, celebrate your good fortune!

Connecting Through a Commercial Service Provider

Connecting to the Internet through a service provider is much the same process as using another's gateway. The service provider builds and maintains the gateway and sells Internet connection access. You choose the way that you want to connect to the service provider. The service provider supplies you with a username and password to connect to its gateway. Service providers usually charge a flat fee to provide a certain amount of Internet access per month or year and a personal e-mail address. Some providers such as America Online (AOL) also offer access to other interesting software or participation in unique discussion groups through their own system.

Ways to Connect to Your Commercial Service Provider

Today there are three main ways to connect your computer to an Internet service provider. The three connection methods are dial-up, DSL, and cable. Each method has its pros and cons. For example, the DSL and cable connection methods are not available to everyone. When choosing a connection type, you can be guided by your own needs, the available choices, and your budget. For example, if you only need e-mail service, then a dial-up connection is probably sufficient. Here is a brief description of each method.

Dial-up Connection

This was the first and probably remains the most common method of connecting to the Internet. Using software that is a normal part of your computer and an inexpensive modem in your computer, you can establish an Internet connection over your telephone line through your Internet service provider (ISP). Your ISP gives you a local telephone number for your computer to call. The dial-up software on your computer makes a telephone call to that number and your modem establishes an Internet connection through the ISP's computer. Most

ISPs charge a flat monthly or yearly fee for unlimited access to the Internet using this method. An advantage to this approach is that you probably have a telephone already and your computer likely has a modem already installed. A drawback is that you lose the normal use of your telephone while you're on the Internet. Another major drawback is that regular telephone lines cannot pass digital information faster than about 22.8 kilobits per second. While that seems like a large number, it strongly limits the speed at which graphical information from the Internet is displayed. And the Internet is hugely graphical!

DSL Connection

To squeeze more speed from regular telephone lines for Internet use, telecommunication companies developed the Digital Subscriber Line (DSL) technology. This technology can allow information to move at speeds of up to 6 megabits per second. Your DSL provider installs a network interface card in your computer, connects it to a DSL modem, and then connects it to your telephone line. As long as your computer is turned on and plugged in, you have an "always on" Internet connection through your telephone line. An advantage, besides the transmission speed, is that you can use your telephone normally even while accessing the Internet. Another advantage is that, unlike a cable connection (see below), you do not share your telephone line with others to access the Internet. The immediate problem with this technology today is that there are distance limitations with DSL. You must be located within a certain distance from your telephone company's internal systems for DSL to work. The only way to find out if DSL is possible for you is to ask a DSL provider (likely a local ISP or your local telephone company). If you are able to have a DSL connection, the monthly charge for the service should be somewhat more than a standard dial-up service.

Cable Connection

The other approach to having fast Internet service uses the coaxial cable that delivers cable television into your home. Cable has the capacity to move a lot of information very quickly—ideal for access to the Internet. Large cable companies are offering Internet service as quickly as they can. A cable company will install a network interface card in your computer, connect it to a cable modem, and then connect the modem to the cable television line in your house. As with the DSL technology, as long as your computer is turned on and plugged in, you have an "always on" Internet connection. An advantage, beyond the speed of Internet access, is that this approach does not affect your telephone in any way. There are several possible problems with this approach, however. For example, you may not have cable television installed in your house or your cable company may not offer Internet access yet. Also, it is possible that, as more people in an area share the service, performance in that area may degrade. The good news is that cable companies are making large investments to address many of these issues. The monthly charge for Internet access is somewhat more than a standard dial-up service and is comparable to the charge for a DSL service.

Future Connection Methods

While the three connection methods described above are the key ones used today, there are new approaches coming to the marketplace. One approach gives you access to the Internet using your television and your cable TV connection but not a computer. By wiring a "WebTV" control box to your television, the Internet is delivered to you without the need for a separate computer. Using a special control, you can send and receive e-mail messages and "surf" the Internet via your television without losing its normal viewing functions. Another approach uses satellite technology to give Internet access to people in remote geographic locations. Those people who are too distant to be physically connected using any of the three main methods will be able to use a small satellite dish to access the Internet, much as people are using satellite television reception today. A third approach is Internet access using cellular phones and other portable wireless information devices. Now people can use e-mail and other Internet facilities as simply as using a telephone. These are just three examples of how the need for Internet access will continue to change the ways in which we are connected.

What to Look for When Choosing an Internet Provider

These are just a few simple guidelines to keep in mind if you want to pursue getting your own Internet connection. Always remember that it is up to you to be an informed buyer. If a provider doesn't have the time or desire to answer your questions before you buy a service, think about the kind of support you are likely to get from that provider when something goes wrong. End of sermon.

There are several basic elements to consider when getting access to the Internet through a provider. First, what kind of computer do you have to work with? Generally, providers are most comfortable supporting PC-compatible computers. The processing power and storage capacity of your computer are also important. Some of the Internet facilities (i.e., World Wide Web) make strong demands on your computer's resources. Be sure to have this information ready for discussion with a service provider.

Second, what is your own level of technical knowledge and comfort when working with your computer? We're not talking nuclear physics here, but it is important to understand that there are many links to this connection chain. You may become involved in levels of technical details that you didn't want to know about. The good news here is that some Internet providers, for a fee, will help you install the connection software on your computer and get it working.

Third, if you are using a dial-up connection, look for a provider with a local telephone number that you use to connect. Some providers also advertise 1-800 numbers that you use. The point here is to avoid additional telephone charges. Without a local number, you end up paying additional costs to a telephone company. It can be a dangerous shock to the system to receive a surprise telephone bill after you've been surfing the Net for 20 hours last month.

Fourth, what is the cost of this connection? Be sure that all the restrictions and assumptions are fully identified. One provider we talked to offered unlimited access to the Internet for a very low monthly charge. The hitch was that you were allowed to be connected for a maximum of only 90 minutes in one stretch. After that, you were automatically disconnected. Of course, you could immediately try to dial back in, but.... This may be perfectly satisfactory for an infrequent e-mail user, but for someone trying to search the Net for information, 90 minutes goes by very quickly (and it usually ends right in the middle of something interesting).

Finally, what kind of technical support does the provider offer? If you have trouble coping now when your computer gives you fits, ask some tough questions about the kind and level of support you can expect from the provider. Also ask about the support policy of the provider (i.e., 24 hours a day, business hours only, etc.).

Security Issues

As always, along with the good things come the not-so-good things. Connecting to the Internet gives others the opportunity to cause trouble for you. There are two kinds of attack on you: direct and indirect.

Hacking or Cracking—Direct Attack

The news today constantly talks about people who break into computer systems. The news reports often call these people *hackers* but, to be strictly correct, these people are *crackers*. *Hacker* is a term that applies to anyone who writes computer program code. *Cracker* is a term that applies to people who use their skills to attempt to access other computers without permission. There are even programs, shared across the Internet, allowing people with less skill to mount an attack.

If you are connected to the Internet, there is the potential for people to *directly* attack your computer. This form of attack is more likely if you have an "always on" connection such as DSL or cable. A dial-up connection is more difficult to attack and is less likely to be attacked. To block these direct attacks, you need something called a *firewall*. This is either a piece of computer hardware or a computer program. If you connect to the Internet indirectly through a network at your workplace, there will probably be a hardware firewall in place. If you connect to the Internet through an ISP, you need to install a commercial *personal firewall program* on your computer. Once installed on your computer, the personal firewall program watches every piece of information that attempts to come or go through your Internet connection. Only legitimate activities that are recognized by the firewall program are allowed to succeed. All other activities are blocked. As new methods of attack are discovered, the firewall manufacturer develops new methods of detecting and blocking them and adds these new methods to the firewall program.

Viruses—Indirect Attack

Even if you are never attacked directly, there are always *indirect* attacks happening through the use of *viruses*. Viruses are small programs that are hidden inside legitimate files or e-mail messages. The virus-infected files might come as part of an e-mail message or might be given to you on a computer disk. When you access these files or e-mail messages, the viruses start running. They are now on the other side of any personal firewall of your computer. The main way to protect against viruses is to install a commercial antivirus program on your computer. These programs will protect your computer from viruses in several ways. They will scan your e-mail messages as you access them, looking for telltale signatures of viruses. They will constantly monitor certain activities of your computer, looking for actions that may signal a virus is starting up. Once a virus is detected, the antivirus program will alert you with a message and guide you in dealing with the virus. As new forms of viruses are discovered, the antivirus program manufacturer develops new methods of detecting and dealing with them and adds these new methods to the antivirus program.

Now that You're Connected and Protected....

Once the physical connection between your computer and the computer of the service provider is made, the service provider will give you an e-mail (electronic mail) address so that you can send and receive e-mail.

E-mail Addresses

All e-mail addresses follow the same format: the person's assigned username followed by the @ symbol, followed by the unique name of the service provider's computer. For example, my university-based e-mail address is

marge@athabascau.ca

In this example, the username portion is **marge** and the unique computer name is **athabascau.ca**. That unique computer name is also called the *domain*. We also have an Internet account with a commercial service provider. That address is

edwardsc@cybersurf.net

In general, an e-mail address has two parts, the username and the domain put together like this:

username@domain

As you probably can guess, that combination needs to be unique on the entire Internet so that the right person receives your important message!

The domain in an e-mail address is actually made up of subdomains, each one separated by a period. In our first example, the domain is **athabascau.ca** and the subdomains, from left to right, are **athabascau** and **ca**. The real way to understand a domain name is to look at the subdomains in it, reading them from right to left. The rightmost subdomain is the most general and the subdomains become more specific as you read to the left. That rightmost subdomain is called the *top-level domain* and there are two different sets of top-level domains: *organizational domains* and *geographical domains*. My two addresses are examples of each style.

In the first example, **marge@athabascau.ca**, the most general subdomain is **ca**. That identifies the computer as being located in Canada (see Table 2.1 for other examples). The next subdomain identifies the university in Canada where the computer is located, **athabascau**. That computer holds a mailbox for a user named **marge**.

The second example, **edwardsc@cybersurf.net**, shows the other kind of domain. Instead of first referring to a geographic location (i.e., **ca** for Canada), the most general part of this domain begins with **net**, identifying this computer system as part of the networking organization domain. Before the days of international networks, the set of organizational domains (Table 2.2) was defined mostly for use in the United States. The next subdomain, **cybersurf**, identifies the name registered on the Internet for a particular company.

Table 2.1. Examples of Geographical Top-Level Domains.

Domain	Meaning
at	Austria
au	Australia
ca	Canada
ch	Switzerland ("Confoederatio Helvetia")
De	Germany ("Deutschland")
Fr	France
Gr	Greece
Jp	Japan
Us	United States

Table 2.2. Examples of Organizational Top-Level Domains.

Domain	Meaning
com	commercial organization
edu	educational institution
gov	government
int	international organization
mil	military
net	networking organization
org	non-profit organization

As a rule, e-mail addresses use all lowercase letters. If you see an address with some uppercase letters, it's safe to change them to lowercase. However, if you decide to use uppercase letters, don't use them on the username as it may make a difference to some computers. The easiest thing to do is to use the exact e-mail address as it was given to you.

The domain in your e-mail address forms the basis for the Internet address of your service provider's computer. This address is called a *Uniform Resource Locator (URL)*.

URLs

The World Wide Web project developed a standard way of referencing an item, whether it was a graphics file, a document, or a link to another computer. This standardized reference is called a URL. The URL is a complete description of the item including its location on the Internet. A typical URL is

http://www.springer-ny.com

The first part of the URL, which ends with the colon, is the protocol that is being used to retrieve the item. In this example, the protocol is HTTP (hypertext transfer protocol), used for the Web. Other protocols are self-evident: gopher for Gopher sites, FTP for FTP sites, and so on. The next part is the domain name of the computer that you need to connect to (**springer-ny.com**). This tells you that the information is on a computer in the commercial top-level domain (**com**). The **springer-ny** indicates that the Web site belongs to the publisher Springer-Verlag in New York. Most Web browsers will automatically add the "http://" if you simply type the other part of the URL, **www.springer-ny.com**

Final Thoughts

To navigate easily around the Web and get to the URL or information you want, you use an application called a *Web browser*. When your ISP initially connects you, it will make sure that your Web browser connects to the Internet. The next chapter describes Web browsers and how to use them effectively.

3
Web Browsers—The View from the Screen

Web Browsers

To access the Web, you will need a Web browser program on your (or your institution's) computer. A Web browser program knows how to interpret and display the hypertext documents that it finds on the Web. There are many browsers on the market. The two most popular graphical user interface (GUI) or Windows-based browsers are *Microsoft Internet Explorer* (Figure 3.1) and *Netscape Communicator* (Figure 3.2).

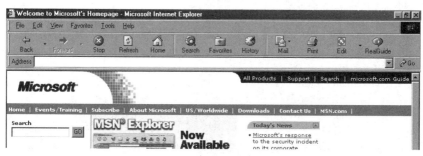

Figure 3.1. Portion of *Internet Explorer* Screen.

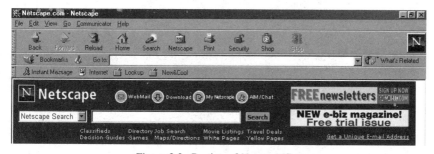

Figure 3.2. Portion of *Netscape* Screen.

Using Web Browsers

When you first start up your Web browser, you will automatically navigate to a Web page that the browser calls its "home" page, which is a Web URL that is initially set by the browser manufacturer or your ISP when it connected you to the Internet. You can navigate to the "home" page of your browser at any time by pressing the browser button called *Home*. In addition to the *Home* button, there are buttons that help you navigate through and display the information you'll find on the Web.

As you navigate to various Web pages, the browsers maintain a small list of the most recently visited Web pages during the current session. The *Forward* and *Back* buttons use this list to allow you to quickly return to Web pages that you have previously viewed in this session.

The *Refresh* or *Reload* button can be pressed to get a complete new copy of the Web page that you are visiting. This is useful if the browser screen reports that the transmission of information has been interrupted or if the display of information appears to be incomplete.

The *Print* button will send a copy of the currently viewed Web page to your printer for hardcopy output. A word of warning: Look for the vertical scroll bar at the right side of the browser window. If that scroll bar is very short in length, it means that the Web page you are viewing has a lot of information on it. This means that printing the currently viewed Web page might result in 30 pages of printed output.

The *Stop* button is used when you realize that you are displaying a Web page that you really didn't want or if the browser has not done what you asked for in a timely manner. Press the *Stop* button to stop the browser from doing whatever it is doing.

Underneath the buttons is a white space called *Address* or *Go To*. This space displays the URL of the Web page you are currently viewing. You can click into this space, delete any URL that is there, type a new URL where you wish to go and press the ENTER or RETURN key on your keyboard. The browser will take you to the URL that you typed. Of course, you can also use hypertext links on the currently viewed Web page to navigate to other sites.

Bookmarks

Bookmarks are a way to collect and organize URLs that you want to remember for future use. The browser either calls them *Bookmarks* or *Favorites*. When you are at a site whose URL you want to remember, click on the *Favorites* or *Bookmarks* button and you can store the URL and the site's title in a file. To return to a site that has been bookmarked, click on the *Bookmarks* or *Favorites* button and then click on the site title and the browser will recall the URL and take you to that site.

Plug-Ins

Technology is changing all the time on the Web. New forms of storing information are being produced constantly. As each new form is created, the creators will also produce browser plug-ins. These are small programs that attach to your browser to display the new storage format. Here's an example from the area of audio. Initially, the only form of storing audio was in a format called wav. Due to its limitations, new forms of storing audio were developed, including a form called MP3. At the same time, browser plug-ins were built to access and play these new forms (MP3 files). When a browser encounters this new form for the first time, it will search its own database for a plug-in that can handle the form. Once it finds the plug-in, the browser will give you directions that will access and attach the plug-in to your browser permanently. You can then access the new form whenever you encounter it again on the Web. Another plug-in that is commonly needed is the Adobe Acrobat Reader for Adobe's *pdf* format files.

Cookies

In an attempt to make your visits to certain Web sites more personal, some sites use the browser to place a small file on your computer that is called a cookie. The next time you visit that Web site, the Web site can retrieve that cookie through the browser to tailor its interaction with you. For example, if you visit a shopping site once, the cookie will contain information about what you were interested in during that visit. When you next visit that site, the Web site will notice that you were interested in shirts and might show you a message about a shirt sale. Generally, you can control whether cookies are created by the browser or not through the Preferences setting in the browser.

Final Thoughts

Now that you are connected to the Internet and protected and your Web browser is enabled, you are ready to take advantage of the two main benefits of the Web: communication and information access.

Part II
Internet-Based Communication

4
Using Electronic Mail (E-mail and Mailing Lists)

Electronic mail (or e-mail) was the first Internet application and is still the most popular one. E-mail is a way of sending messages between people or computers through networks of computer connections. E-mail is not limited to just the Internet. E-mail messages can be moved through gateways to other networks and systems, such as Compuserve or America Online. Many businesses already have an internal e-mail system and, with a little work by the employer, employees can send and receive messages from other businesses via the Internet.

E-mail on the Internet is analogous to the regular postal system but faster in delivery of mail. E-mail combines a word processor function and a post office function in one program. Here's a typical scenario. You start up your e-mail program and use a command to begin a new message. You type the message and identify the recipient's e-mail address and your return address. Then, you "send" your message; this is something like dropping your letter in the regular postbox. The electronic post office in your system takes over and passes your message on. Electronic packets of data carry your message toward its ultimate destination mailbox. Your message will often have to pass through a series of intermediate networks to reach the recipient's address. Since networks can and do use different e-mail formats, a gateway at each network will translate the format of your e-mail message into one that the next network understands. Each gateway also reads the destination address of your message and sends the message on in the direction of the destination mailbox. The routing choice takes into consideration the size of your message and also the amount of traffic on various networks. Because of this routing, it will take varying amounts of times to send messages from you to the same person. On one occasion, it might be only a few minutes; on others, it might be a few hours. This can be compared to the situation of taking an airplane to travel from New York to San Francisco at different times. Depending on the amount of passenger traffic at the time that you decide to go, you may be able to take a direct flight with no stops or you may have to be routed from New York to Chicago to Denver to San Francisco. Either way you get to your destination, one route just takes longer than the other.

When your message reaches its destination, the recipient can read the message, respond to you with just a few key strokes, forward your message to someone else, file it, print it, or delete it.

Anatomy of an E-mail Message

E-mail messages will always have several features in common regardless of the program used to create the e-mail. A typical e-mail message includes a "From:" line with the sender's electronic address, a date and time line, a "To:" line with the recipient's electronic address, a "Subject:" line, and the body of the message. If there are any spelling or punctuation mistakes in the recipient's address, the message will be sent back to you from the electronic post office. The "Subject:" line is the place to give a clear, one-line description of your message. This description is usually displayed when someone checks their e-mail. Then they can decide how quickly they want to read your message!

Many mail programs can automatically attach a signature line at the end of your message. The signature line can include the sender's name, telephone number, postal address, and Internet address. This function can be turned on or off.

Figure 4.1 contains a sample e-mail message. The format may vary on your system, but the general idea will be the same. In the example, the first line starts with the word "From." This line shows the userid of the person or computer that sent the message. In this case it was **marge@cs.athabascau.ca**.

The "Subject" line tells the recipient what the message is about. Make your subject lines very clear because, when a recipient has dozens of messages, the subject line description is often the basis for deciding what is read first!

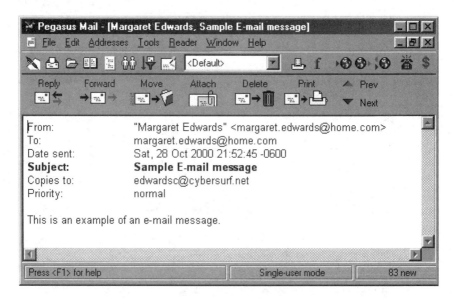

Figure 4.1. A Sample E-mail Message.

The "To:" line indicates the address to which the message was sent. In the example, the message was sent to our commercial Internet address. If the message had been sent to other people at the same time, their addresses would also appear on this line.

The fourth line is a date/time stamp of when the message was sent. The time will include either a time zone designation (Mountain Daylight Time) or GMT (Greenwich Mean Time) when a standard time reference is needed.

If the message has been copied to others, their addresses will appear on the "Copies to:." Copying or forwarding messages to others is easy to do with most mail programs. For this reason, be very prudent in what you say in a message. You never know where it will end up because you have no control over the message once you have sent it. It is possible to also send "blind" copies of this message to other people. The other recipients of the message won't know that these additional copies have been sent.

Next comes the body of the message. While most e-mail messages are text, if your computer and the recipient's computer have the facilities, you can send data files, sound, and visual images via e-mail. In the next section we will outline some of the legal issues surrounding e-mail message contents and discuss some standards of Internet etiquette.

Legal Issues

Privacy, libel, and copyright are legal issues that can affect e-mail users. Understand that privacy is *not* assured with electronic mail. There are no legal requirements that prevent an institution or company from reading incoming and outgoing e-mail messages. If you are using your employer's equipment, this is especially applicable. In addition, once you have sent a message, you have no control over what the recipient may do. He may send a copy to someone else without your knowledge. Also, don't assume that messages you receive are private. The sender may have sent that same message to others without using the "Copies to:" function. A final note about privacy: even though you have deleted a mail message from your mailbox, don't assume that it has been completely erased. Many institutional and company policies require regular backups of their computer system disks, which generally hold incoming and outgoing mail messages. It is possible that a copy of your message was taken during a regular system backup. Be aware that your e-mail records can be subpoenaed.

A second legal issue for e-mail users is libel. Libel is applicable within e-mail messages and newsgroups (see Chapter 5). Take care with your comments. What you say can be held against you.

Finally, copyright law applies to transferring files and information. It is illegal to distribute copyrighted information by any means, including electronic transfer. It is not uncommon to find material that has been scanned by a user for personal use and then distributed through e-mail. Unless the copyright owner has granted specific permission for the transfer of such material, it is illegal to do so.

E-mail Etiquette

Many of the people who you communicate with over the Internet will never meet you. Their impressions about you will come entirely from the tone, style, and content of your messages. There are several rules of the road for using the Information Highway.

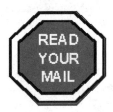

Many people don't have a regular routine of reading their e-mail. This allows messages to build up, often at a great rate! When you finally do sit down to read your e-mail, you may have hundreds of messages. Not only is this taxing on you, it is rude to the senders of those messages. You may miss something important by not keeping up with your mail. If you are getting mail that you don't want, inform the senders that you want your name taken off their distribution list.

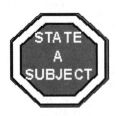

When sending messages, always include a clear description of the message on the subject line. This practice is great for helping you to crystallize your thoughts and express your key idea clearly at the beginning of your message. This courtesy allows recipients to prioritize the order in which they read and respond to their e-mail. It also keeps you from long, run-on messages that have people asking, "What was the question again?"

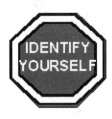

Don't assume that the recipient of your message can figure out who you are from the information in the "From:" line. Be sure to give any contact information that you want the recipient to have. Some people copy a short standard personal identification file into their messages to make this easier, i.e., a signature line.

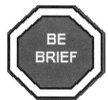

E-mail messages often tend to be "stream of consciousness" based. They ramble on as you try to put your thoughts together while you are responding. Take time to organize your messages or responses before you begin to enter them. Your recipients will appreciate the succinctness of your messages. This will help build you a positive Internet reputation.

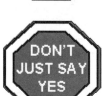

Nothing is more frustrating than receiving an e-mail message that just says "Yes." You're left wondering which of the six questions you originally posed is being answered. You know how that makes you feel, so don't do it to others. Always include, in a brief form, the question to which you're replying.

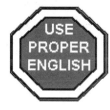

A message full of spelling and punctuation errors reflects badly on you. Ensure that your e-mail messages are properly spelled, punctuated and grammatically correct. This may be the only time that people "see" you. Be sure to make a good impression. For convenience, there are a number of widely used abbreviations found in Internet communications, including

Abbreviation	Meaning
BTW	By The Way
IMHO	In My Humble Opinion
TIA	Thanks in advance
FWIW	For What It's Worth

For a more complete list of abbreviations, check Computing Corner at **www.computingcorner.com/help/emoticons/emailabb.htm**

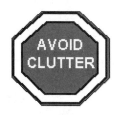

When replying to a message, unless it is really necessary, avoid including the previous message. The Information Highway is often backlogged with volumes of unnecessary information. Don't contribute to this cluttering problem. In the same way, avoid copying the message to a long list of users who are either marginally interested or completely uninterested in what you are sending. Also avoid including a request for automatic confirmation of receipt of the message unless it is vital to have one. Since many mailing packages require only a quick click of the mouse to request confirmation of receipt and then confirmation of reading, users get carried away checking off these and many other unnecessary options. The result is several "confirming" messages being sent for every one real message. Unless the message is urgent, avoid tagging it as such.

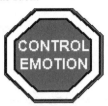

Although e-mail allows easy expression of ideas, it does not allow the recipient of your message to hear the tone of your voice or see the body language that accompanies your message. Be careful, for example, in how you express anger through your message. Because e-mail is faceless, many people seem to lose their inhibitions and feel that they can say exactly what they want (but probably shouldn't!). Angry blasts meant for one person are often forwarded to others and used against you. Often in written messages it's difficult to identify humor or sarcasm. Use a "smiley" to convey your emotions. Smileys are an example of "emoticons," icons for indicating emotions. Turn your head sideways to see them: :-) (Happy Smiley), :-((Sad Smiley), or 8-) (Smiley with glasses). There's got to be a bit of fun in all this serious message-sending! For a larger list of possibilities , look at EFF's (Extended) Guide to the Internet at **http://www.eff.org/papers/eegtti/eeg_286.html** And finally, DON'T SHOUT. Typing your message in all capital letters is like shouting. Use capital letters SPARINGLY, only for emphasis.

Mailing Lists

Mailing lists are an extension of e-mail. When you send an e-mail message to someone, you indicate his or her address. When you consistently want to mail to the same group of people, you can set up a special recipient name called an *alias*. For example, a hospital could create an alias called "nursing" that lists the e-mail addresses of all the directors of nursing. To send a message to all the directors of nursing, you simply specify "nursing" in the "To:" line and the same message will be sent to everyone on that list (alias). The directors of nursing can use this method to have an electronic discussion group. One director sends a message about a certain topic that is distributed to all those users identified by the alias "nursing" (all the other directors of nursing). When another director wants to respond to the topic, a message is sent again to "nursing," and all the directors of nursing receive it.

A mailing list is like an alias that contains hundreds or thousands of users from all over the Internet. Any message sent to the mailing list "alias" will automatically be sent to everyone on the mailing list. Everything that anyone says through the mailing list goes to everyone on the mailing list. Mailing lists facilitate electronic discussion groups. Each mailing list resides at a specific computer and is looked after by a human administrator. The host computer is responsible for distributing incoming messages to all mailing list members. The administrator is responsible for maintaining the mailing list. Some mailing lists are also moderated. In these lists, there is a moderator who reviews each incoming message for appropriateness and either passes it through for distribution or rejects it. Some moderators will also prepare *digests*, something like an issue of a magazine. The digest will be a whole set of messages and articles in one package, making it much easier to keep up with the messages.

These mailing lists are maintained in two ways, either manually by a person or by a program. In the manual approach, the list administrator takes care of adding or deleting addresses from the master distribution list. In the program approach, you send messages to the address of a computer that provides this service. The most common mailing list administration program is called *Listserv* (standing for **List server**). Many of the mailing lists in our catalogue are maintained by "Listserv" systems. We'll describe the ways of subscribing and unsubscribing to mailing lists in the next section.

Subscribing, Unsubscribing, and Mailing to Mailing Lists

Mailing lists are traditionally organized around specific topics. Many of these are profession or occupation-specific. For example, NURSENET is a mailing list that hosts general discussion about nursing. Other examples of profession-specific mailing lists include GradNrse, MEDLAB-L (for Medical Laboratory Technology), and Psychiatric Nursing List. These and others of interest to health care professionals are found in Appendix 2.

As we described in the previous section, mailing lists are administered either by a person or by a program. In either case, you subscribe or unsubscribe to a list by sending an e-mail message to a specific address. This address will be for the administrator of the list, whether human or machine. The format for most subscribe/unsubscribe messages to a list administrator follows a similar format.

As an example, to subscribe to NURSENET, you send an e-mail message to LISTSERV@LISTSERV.UTORONTO.CA. By the address, you can see that this is an automated list (the address LISTSERV gives it away). For subscribe and unsubscribe messages, the "Subject:" line is ignored so you don't put anything in it. However, in the body of the message, you must put, on a line by itself, the command

SUB NURSENET <first name> <last name>

where the <first name> and <last name> are your first and last names. After a period of time, you'll receive a confirmation message that you are subscribed. Shortly after that, you'll begin receiving messages from the list. You can unsubscribe in the same way with the UNSUB command, but you don't have to enter your name. The line in the body would look like

UNSUB NURSENET

Listserv machines have other commands to give you control of the messages you receive. To get a list of available commands, send a message to the Listserv machine with the word HELP, on a line by itself, in the body of the message. A return message will give you a complete command set.

Once you have subscribed to any of these lists, you will receive instruction on what address to send messages to if you want those messages "posted to the list" (i.e., have a copy of your message sent to all addresses on the mailing list).

Finding a Mail List

Mailing lists are scattered across the Web. One place to go to look for a comprehensive collection of mailing lists is **www.liszt.com**. This site supports searching and provides some information about the lists.

Mailing List Etiquette

There are a few additional points of etiquette that apply to mailing lists specifically. Most of them have to do with reducing the amount of unnecessary messages on the Net. It is important to remember that the resources of the Internet are not infinite. If people on the Net do not take responsibility for "conserving the environment," so to speak, all users will suffer.

The first point is common sense. When you first get on the Net, it is very tempting to join many different mailing lists because they all sound so interesting. That's true. They *are* interesting, and hundreds of people read them and respond daily. But the number of messages generated from even one mailing list can be overwhelming. Try joining mailing lists one at a time. Monitor how much information comes from a list and whether you really want to be on this list. As we said earlier, you need to have the time to read your mail, so choose your lists carefully.

Once you've joined a mailing list, spend some time *lurking*. Lurking means just listening in on the group discussion without replying. This will allow you to discover the tone of the group, the types of topics covered, and current topics of conversation. Asking questions or making comments immediately upon joining a group, without knowing the culture, can result in angry censoring by the group. One of the most important sources for topics and the purpose of the list can be found in the FAQ (Frequently Asked Questions). It is a list of questions and answers that is regularly posted on a list to help newcomers understand what this particular list is all about. Find it on your list and read it.

A sure sign of a newcomer is a message sent to the list "just to see if it works." Even though the subject line may say "Test message, please ignore," it can still annoy a lot of people. Don't forget that a message posted to the list means that message is sent to *all* the addresses on the list.

Along that same thought, be careful in how you respond to a question that someone posts to the list. You may have an answer, but it is better to send that answer in a message to the *person* who asked the question rather than post the answer to the list. If several people respond to the originator, it is more efficient and effective for the originator to summarize the answers and post them once to the list.

Finally, we want to reinforce the importance of how you present yourself through your messages. When you send a message to friends, they will make allowances for you because they know you. When hundreds of people all over the world are reading your responses, take the time to use correct spelling, punctuation, and grammar. Present yourself well! Someday you may meet some of these people face to face.

5
Newsgroups

Discussions take place on the Internet using both mailing lists and newsgroups, but there is a significant difference between the two methods. A mailing list discussion comes directly to your electronic mailbox, just like a letter is delivered by a postal service. However, the messages that form discussions in newsgroups are only sent to the newsgroup administrator, who then sends them to Internet newsgroup system sites (not individual subscribers). You then read the messages in the newsgroup at a particular system site just as you would walk down the hall to read the messages posted on a bulletin board. In fact, the origin of newsgroups was as a bulletin board service where messages could be posted for all to see. In summary, instead of the messages coming directly to you via a mailing list, you go to a place where the messages are posted in a newsgroup and read them there.

What Is Usenet?

Usenet (User's Network) is made up of all the machines that receive network newsgroups. A machine that receives these newsgroups is called a Usenet server. Any computer system that wants to carry newsgroups of interest to that site can be a Usenet server. If you are affiliated with an institution, it is probably a Usenet site. Ask your system administrator! If you have your own Internet access through a service provider, ask that provider about the newsgroups that it carries.

Instead of forwarding all messages to all users on a mailing list, Usenet forwards all messages (called *articles* to keep up the newspaper analogy) not to individual subscribers, but to other Usenet servers who forward them on until all machines that are part of Usenet have a copy of your article (message). Individuals then use programs called "newsreaders" to access the newsgroup through their own computer.

A typical Usenet server receives more than 20,000 articles per day. To organize all these articles, they are assigned to specific newsgroups. Newsgroups are further collected into hierarchies, similar to the domains described in relation to e-mail addresses. Table 5.1 shows an example of some of the most important Usenet newsgroup hierarchies.

Table 5.1. Example of Usenet Newsgroup Hierarchies.

Name	Topic
alt	alternative newsgroups
bionet	biology
biz	business, marketing, advertisements
comp	computers
k12	kindergarten to grade 12
misc	anything that doesn't fit into another category
news	about Usenet itself
rec	recreation, hobbies, the arts
sci	science of all types

Every Usenet server subscribes to specific newsgroups. Not all newsgroups are available on all Usenet servers. Again, you will have to ask your system administrator or service provider for a list of newsgroups to which your system subscribes.

Some newsgroups are moderated. This means that you cannot post articles directly to the newsgroup. Instead, all messages sent to this newsgroup will be automatically routed to the volunteer moderator. The moderator then decides what articles to send on to the newsgroup. Articles may be edited by the moderator or grouped with other articles before they are forwarded to the newsgroup. In some cases, the moderator may decide not to forward an article at all. Moderators exist to limit the number of low-quality articles in a newsgroup, especially all those "me too" or "I agree" type of articles.

Components of a Usenet Article

Messages sent to a newsgroup are called articles. Just like an e-mail message, all articles have common features. Each article begins with a header. The header, which may be up to twenty lines long, contains technical information about the article. The body of the article follows. The same rules of the road that we discussed in Chapter 4 apply when sending articles to Usenet newsgroups. Finally, a signature block is placed at the end of your article. Although your name will appear in the header, a signature block with at least your name and e-mail address is standard. Many users place quotations or small graphics on their signature line.

In Figure 5.1, you can see that there are individual articles (e.g., "Acid Reflux") and that the moderator has grouped some articles together (e.g., "Bad Breath"). The numbers in the square brackets tell you how long the individual article is (i.e., "Acid Reflux" is 10 lines long) or how many articles are in each group (i.e., "Bad Breath" has five articles). The name of this newsgroup is **misc.kids.health**.

misc.kids.health			
📄 "The perfect food"	[44]	04/05	Bryan J. M
📄 Acid Reflux	[10]	04/04	Ken Solon
📄 Atrial Septal Defect -- Anybody been throu	[20]	04/04	Lenore Ma
📁 Bad Breath	[5]		
📁 Chicken Pox Twice in a Month	[4]		
📁 goomy eyes	[2]		
📁 Growing up connected to nature	[3]		
📄 gummy eyes	[8]	04/05	Laura Joh
📄 Labial adhesions	[18]	04/05	Nancy@dι

Figure 5.1. Example of Articles Found in a Newsgroup.

Joining a Newsgroup

When you first join or subscribe to a newsgroup, it is advisable to initially spend time *lurking* (discussed in Chapter 4). You will want to monitor the articles in the group for a while to see what the tone of the group is (are the articles academic in tone or informal?), who the regular participants are, and what types of topics are discussed. Most news groups have an FAQ (Frequently Asked Questions) file that is well worth reading before you start asking questions that will reflect badly on you!

Another resource to explore is a Web page for new users of Usenet found at **www.landfield.com/faqs/by-newsgroup/news/news.announce.newusers.html**

Articles that appear on this Web page include

- rules for posting to Usenet
- how to work with the Usenet community
- FAQs about Usenet
- Emily Postnews on Netiquette
- Writing style for Usenet

Reading Articles

To read the articles posted to a newsgroup, you use a program called a newsreader. A newsreader is the interface to Usenet that allows you to choose the newsgroups to which you wish to belong, or select and display articles. Using a newsreader, you can also save articles to a file, mail a copy to someone else, or print them. Responding to the article's author or the newsgroup is also done through the newsreader program. Web browsers have a built-in newsreader.

Posting Articles

After you've been lurking for a while, you will decide that you have something to say to the newsgroup to which you've subscribed. Before you reply to an article, determine if your response would be best sent to the author of the previous article or to the entire newsgroup.

Once you've decided where to direct your message, your specific newsreader program will have a number of functions to assist you in sending your own article. Again, as these functions vary with the newsreader program, we will not list them all here, but rather direct you to the documentation provided for your system's newsreader.

Don't try a test message to the newsgroup. The people who spent valuable time and money to download your file that says "This is a test" will be less than amused with you and may send unpleasant remarks your way! There are several newsgroups designed to test whether or not your messages are getting through: **misc.test** and **alt.test**. When these newsgroups receive a posting from you, they will automatically send a reply to tell you that you were successful in sending your article. Use these newsgroups to perfect your article-sending skills first.

Final Thoughts

Newsgroups and mailing lists exemplify the power of the Net. You have the ability to call on the resources and creativity of people around the world to help you. As well, you can contribute your experience and share your knowledge with others. This borderless Global Village is the true spirit of the Internet.

6
Internet Chat

Mailing Lists and Newsgroups enable asynchronous or time-independent discussions on the Internet. Participants can post and read messages at any time. They don't have to be taking part in the discussion at the same time. "Live" or synchronous discussion is accomplished through either Internet Relay Chat (IRC) or Web-based Chat. Both approaches use the same underlying technology but have different appearances. To use IRC, for example, you type commands to connect to an IRC server or hold conversations with other people. For Web-based Chat, you use your Web browser to navigate to a chat room and click on buttons to join the conversations. For the purposes of this book, we are focusing on Web-based Chat. For fuller information on IRC, look at **http://www.mirc.com/irc.html**.

Chat Rooms

Chat rooms provide a way for you to "talk" with anyone who is present in the chat room at the same time. Chat rooms (sometimes called channels) generally have a specific theme such as women's health, senior's health, or endometriosis. There are also chat rooms organized by professional practice discipline or area of practice such as medical technologists or emergency. There are no directories of chat rooms. To find a chat room related to a specific topic, you would use a Web search engine (see Chapters 7 and 8). Once you have identified a chat room, you'll want to determine whether the discussion is moderated or unmoderated.

There are two types of chat rooms: moderated and unmoderated. In the moderated chat room, a person, often a volunteer, acts as host for the chat. This person is responsible for keeping the discussion on track and for removing offensive or unruly participants. Some moderated chat rooms use keyword filtering software to eliminate offensive language from the conversations. Many moderated chat rooms have topics scheduled on a weekly basis so that you know what time to join in for a particular topic of interest.

Unmoderated chat rooms have no one monitoring them, and so anything can be and often is said. These unmoderated chats are very disappointing for people

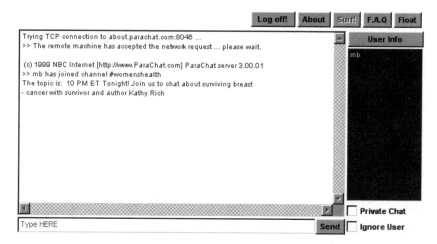

Figure 6.1. Example of a Web-based chat room.

truly seeking information and support for a variety of topics listed under health on some of the more common index sites. Instead of helpful information, they find an unending stream of profanity and pornography. Stay with moderated chat rooms for the best discussions!

Once you have identified a chat room and gone to the site, you will have to sign up and select a username and sometimes a password. The name that you select provides some degree of privacy provided you select a name that does not identify you. Be aware that, because you can't verify the identity of others in the chat room, participants may take on identities or personas very different from their real selves. Once you have joined the chat room, you will see a split screen as in Figure 6.1.

On the left side of the screen, you will see a box that contains the ongoing discussion. Underneath this main area is a box in which you type your text and a button to send it. For the sake of the flow of conversation, make your comments short and to the point. The box on the right, lists the names of those in the chat room. Most chat rooms will announce when someone joins or leaves the conversation. A chat room is often like being in a room full of people—there are many conversations going on at the same time. If there are many people in a chat room, it is often difficult to follow the simultaneous discussions. Many chat rooms allow you to send a private message to another person in the chat room, without everyone else seeing it.

Safe Chatting

Before you begin to participate in chat rooms, some words of caution:

- As mentioned before, when selecting a screen name, don't use your username or other information by which you could be identified. While the majority of people you meet in chat rooms will be innocuous, there will always be some people to stay clear of. It's almost impossible, from the information that you glean from chatting, to tell the "good guys" from the "bad guys," so don't let your guard down!
- Each time you join a chat room, lurk for a time before contributing any comments. Try to pick up the threads of the various conversations that are going on before "speaking."
- Many chat rooms post codes of conduct that require appropriate behaviors and respectful conversations. If inappropriate behaviors or disrespectful comments are being posted to the chat room, go somewhere else or try again another time.
- Never give out personal information such as your telephone number, address, workplace, passwords, or computer information.
- There have been many tragic stories in the media about unfortunate face-to-face meetings between people who initially met through the Internet. Use extreme caution and lots of common sense if you plan to meet a new "cyberpal" in person.

Part III
Internet-Based Information Access

7
Search Engines and Beyond

Each one of the more than 1 billion Web pages and the additional 1 million pages added each month have a unique URL. Finding what you want in that sea of information can be daunting. Search sites are the answer to finding the information "needle" in the WWW "haystack"!

Search sites bring millions of hypertext pages, with their images and multimedia elements into an orderly and searchable structure. Software agents or "spiders" are sent out by search sites to electronically "crawl" the Web, collecting home pages, keywords, and abstracts that are used to build indexes and directories that can be searched. Search sites use both indexes and directories (sometimes called search engines) to manage Internet information. You can go to any search engine or Web index by typing the URL in the textbox of your Web browser. Once at the site, you begin the search for information by typing a key word or phrase in the textbox. Chapter 8 outlines a variety of strategies and techniques for refining your search. This chapter discusses the various types of search sites and gives some examples.

Once you type in the keyword, the search is performed and the results displayed on your screen. The results will be in the form of hypertext links that allow you to click on your choice and be automatically connected with the selected site. Some of the search sites provide a "degree of relevance" for each site found. This gives you a sense of how closely matched the site is to the keyword or phase that you used. The more specific the keyword or phrase, the more likely it is that the results will be useful. Once you are acquainted with the types of search sites, you can choose the site most appropriate to your needs.

Web Indexes

Web indexes are massive, computer-generated databases containing specific information related to millions of Web pages and/or Usenet newsgroup articles. The key to understanding indexes is that they are totally a computer-based approach to collecting and categorizing information. These indexes are continually updated. They can be searched for the specific information you need. Classic Web indexes are *AltaVista Search* (**www.altavista.digital.com**),

Hot-Bot (**www.hotbot.com**), *Open Text Index* (**index.opentext.net**), and *World Wide Web Worm* (**www.cs.colorado.edu/wwww**).

Alta Vista (**www.altavista.com**) is one of the largest search engines. It does require some understanding of Boolean search terms (see Chapter 8), but does return excellent results for finely tuned search terms. Less specific search terms, however, will generate an overload of generally unwanted sites.

Web Directories

Web directories are lists of Web sites linked by hypertext, and hierarchically organized into categories by topic and subtopic. People, not just computers, create Web directories. Web directories often contain reviews or recommendations of sites. Because people review the sites, Web directories cover fewer sites than Web indexes but the quality and kind of information is often better. Web directories can also be searched. *Yahoo!* (**www.yahoo.com**) and *Magellan Internet Guide* (**www.mckinley.com**) are directories.

Open Directory (**www.dmoz.org**) is a Web directory that relies on volunteers, not automated "spiders," to create a massive directory of what is available on the Web. Volunteers collect lists of Web sites under specific categories and then maintain those categories by removing URLs that stop being valid and adding new ones in their place. This generally results in higher quality search results since the directory information is constantly being reviewed. Open Directory is included in searches by a variety of search engines such as Lycos and Hot Bot.

Other Types of Search Engines

Excite (**www.excite.com**), *Go.com* (**www.go.com**), *Lycos* (**www. lycos.com**), and *WebCrawler* (**www.webcrawler.com**) are hybrids. They offer both heavy-duty Web indexes and Web directories.

Google (**www.google.com**) uses its own search technology to rank search terms more intelligently, not only by how often they appear, but by whether or not they pertain to other information on the particular Web site. This means that the results make more sense, for example, scarlet fever (the disease) versus Scarlet Fever (the high school newspaper.)

Choosing a Search Engine

If you know the specific topic that you want to find, then you can use a keyword search through one of the indexes or hybrids (see Figures 7.1 and 7.2 for an example search).

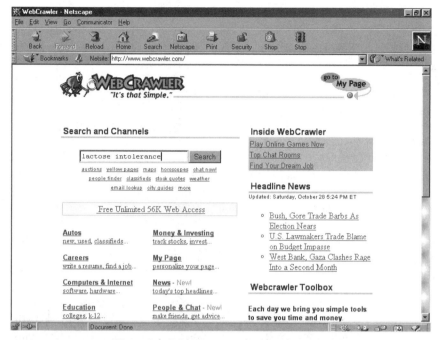

Figure 7.1. Initiating a search using *WebCrawler*.

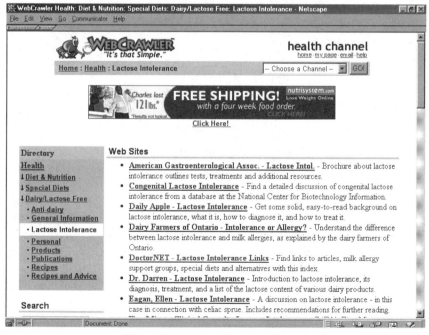

Figure 7.2. Results of *WebCrawler* search.

However, if you're not looking for a specific piece of information, but rather want to browse a topic area, then a directory will allow you to drill down through subdirectories to narrow your search. See Figures 7.3 and 7.4 for an example.

When you want the most comprehensive search possible, you can use a Metasearch site. Metasearch sites load your search request (keyword search) simultaneously into many different indexes and directories. MetaCrawler (**www.metacrawler.com**), for example, simultaneously submits your search to nine different search engines. Dogpile (**www.dogpile.com**) searches other search engines, Usenet discussion groups, and other Internet areas.

There is no single best search site or approach because your needs vary each time you want to find information on the Internet. In the examples above, it is very efficient to use a search site to locate very specific material related to lactose intolerance. However, if you just want to see what the Internet has to offer in an area such as nutrition, it may be much more profitable and efficient to use a directory and follow the links, or consult a catalogue such as the one provided in Appendix 1.

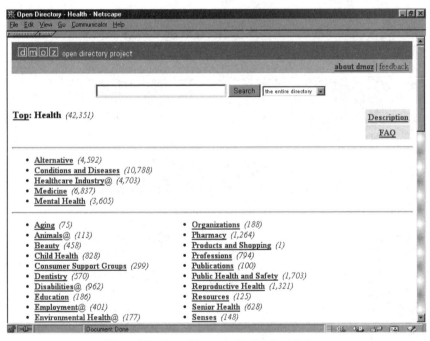

Figure 7.3. *Open Directory Project* health directory.

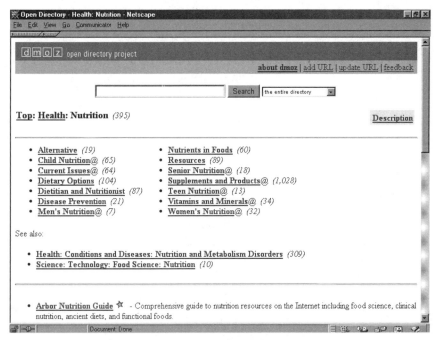

Figure 7.4. *Open Directory Project* health subtopics.

Final Thoughts

As the Internet grows in popularity and its use becomes more a part of our lives, you can expect to see more tools developed to make it easier to locate the valuable information that is out there on the Net. In the meantime, the tools described in this chapter will help you discover the power and value of the Net.

8
Search Strategies and Techniques

Initiating an Internet search for information is very simple and very complex. It's simple because you just type a keyword or phrase into the textbox of the search engine and press the *ENTER* key. The complexity comes when the search returns a list of 62,000 Web sites containing the keyword! There are several techniques that can be used to refine a search to identify sites that truly meet your information needs.

Search Terms

It is essential to select search terms that accurately reflect the information for which you are searching. For example, to find information about why dairy products bothered my sister, I did a search on Google (**www.google.com**) using the keywords *milk allergy*. Figure 8.1 illustrates the results.

The topic *milk allergy* is a very broad subject area and, as a result, the search engine returns a large number of "hits" or Web sites that match the keywords. One strategy to refine the search results is to use synonyms or related terms in your search. They will often yield different results. (Be aware also that if you capitalize a word of text in your search term, only sites that have that same capitalization will be returned. Lower-case words are matched independently of case.) Figure 8.2 illustrates the results of using the alternate keywords *lactose intolerance*.

Search engines will automatically insert an AND between words in a search term. So the search in Figure 8.2 was done for the words *lactose* and *intolerance* anywhere on the same Web page. The returned sites are not necessarily related to the subject of lactose intolerance but definitely contain both words somewhere on the Web page. To be more specific in your search, make the keywords into a phrase by enclosing them in quotation marks. Figure 8.3 illustrates the results of a search for *"lactose intolerance"* (note the quotation marks).

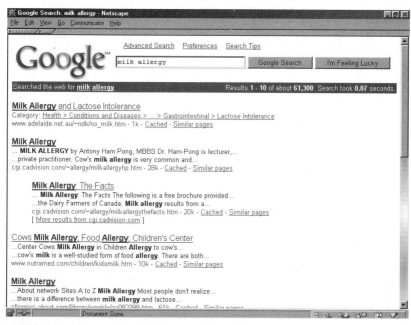

Figure 8.1. Search results for keywords *milk allergy*

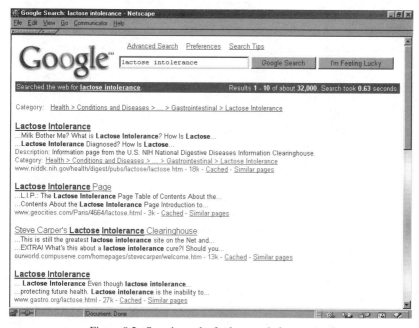

Figure 8.2. Search results for keywords *lactose intolerance*.

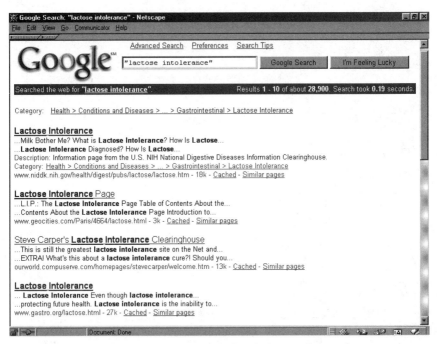

Figure 8.3. Search results for "*lactose intolerance*."

The difference in the number of results between Figure 8.2 and 8.3 illustrates the further refinement that is brought to the search by using a phrase for the search term, not just keywords.

Many Web sites will also have a "search" facility for the site itself. This helps you to further refine a search once you know that the site has the type of information you are seeking. The site-specific search just helps to know where on the site to actually find the information that you want.

Advanced Searching

Most search engines coach you in advanced searching techniques so you don't have to learn about Boolean logic to use them. Boolean logic uses operators such as AND, OR, and NOT to include or exclude items from the search. Many search engines also allow you to put a + (plus sign) in front of terms to be included and a – (minus sign) in front of terms to be excluded from the search. Figure 8.4 illustrates the use of an *Advanced Search* from the Google search engine. In this example, by filling in the blanks, you don't have to know where to use plus signs, quotes, or AND operators. In our search, we're looking for the phrase *lactose intolerance*. We have excluded information about *infant* and *child*. We have also excluded *.com* (commercial) Web sites, because we're not looking for product information. The search also specifies English-only results.

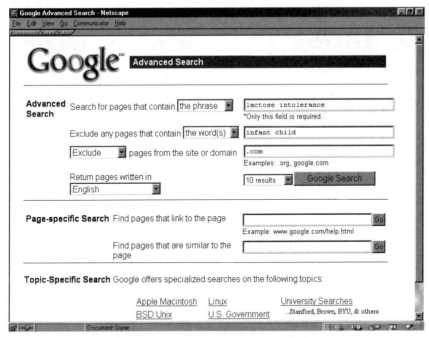

Figure 8.4. Example of an advanced search screen.

Figure 8.5 illustrates the results of the advanced search. If you look in the textbox at the top of the results screen, you will see that the search engine has automatically added the quotation marks around the words *lactose intolerance*, added a minus sign before each of the words *infant* and *child*, and has also added a special term *–sites:.com* to exclude the commercial Web sites from the search. Notice how adding the restrictions on infant, child, .com sites, and English-only has dramatically reduced the number of hits. Remember we started our search using the words *milk allergy* and got 61,300 hits. By using various refinements in our search, we're down to 4,910 hits. This is still a large number of sites to investigate, but you can continue to refine the search and look for specific items of interest such as recipes, support groups, symptom lists, and diagnostic procedures by adding more search terms. The point is that the more specific you make your search request, the more usable your search results will be.

Most search engines will allow you to use the wildcard symbol * (asterisk) in the search term. The asterisk tells the search engine to report on Web sites that partially match the search term. This can be useful if you want to catch alternate spellings or truncations of your search term. For example, you can find Web pages with information on lactose intolerance by using the search term *lacto**. As another example, using the search term *child** ensures that you find Web pages with any of the words *child*, *children*, or *childhood*. However, use this wildcard approach appropriately. As you can see in Figure 8.6, we may have gotten hits on lactose intolerance by using the search term *lacto**, but we also found kebob sauce and ovo-lacto vegetarian recipes.

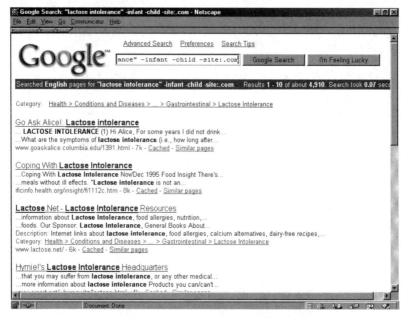

Figure 8.5. Search results for advanced search options.

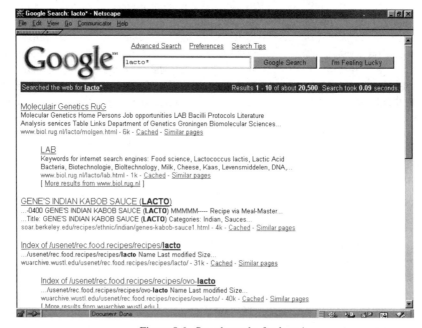

Figure 8.6. Search results for *lacto**.

Final Thoughts

There are no best search engines or foolproof techniques for finding information on the Internet. As you explore the Internet, you will develop your own preferences for which search engines to use, depending on the type of information you are seeking. The more you experiment with search strategies, the more experienced you will become at refining the search to find the information you want.

9
Using and Citing Information from the Internet

Using Information from the Internet

The Internet is a wide-open frontier. Anyone, for the cost of a homepage, can put any type of information on the Internet. Therefore, a note of caution is necessary. All information on the Internet is not created equal. You must use your judgment in determining the validity and reliability of information that you find on the Internet. Sites that are moderated or sponsored by educational institutions, national/international associations, or governments tend to provide more credible information. However, there are also some excellent personal sites, so your discernment is the key to using only credible information. If a site asks you to pay to see the information it provides, this should sound a cautionary note. Certainly you will have to pay to subscribe to services such as database searching through MEDLINE or CINAHL Direct, but a subscription such as this differs from the cyber snake oil that awaits the unwary. Two initiatives that give some guidance to evaluating health information found on the Internet warrant mention.

Health Summit Working Group Evaluation Criteria

A Health Summit Working Group convened by Mitretek Systems' Health Information Technology Institute has developed a set of criteria for evaluating health information on the Internet. These criteria were developed as a result of three summit meeting held between 1996 and 1998. Members of the working group that developed the criteria included health care providers, medical librarians, information resources experts, and consumers. The report and full discussion of the criteria can be found at **http://hitiweb.mitretek.org/docs/policy.html** . Table 9.1 outlines the criteria developed by this group.

Table 9.1. Criteria for evaluating health information on the Internet developed by the health summit working group.

Credibility	Includes the source, currency, relevance/utility, and editorial review process for the information
Content	Must be accurate and complete, and an appropriate disclaimer provided.
Disclosure	Includes informing the user of the purpose of the site, as well as any profiling or collection of information associated with using the site
Links	Evaluated according to selection, architecture, content, and back linkages
Design	Encompasses accessibility, logical organization (navigability), and internal search capability
Interactivity	Includes feedback mechanisms and means for exchange of information among users
Caveats	Clarification of whether site function is to market products and services or is a primary information content provider

Health On the Net (HON) Code of Conduct

The Health On the Net Foundation has elaborated the Code of Conduct to help standardize the reliability of medical and health information available on the World Wide Web. The HONcode is not an award system, nor does it intend to rate the quality of the information provided by a Web site. It only defines a set of principles to hold Web site developers to basic ethical standards in the presentation of information and to help make sure readers always know the source and the purpose of the data they are reading. Each site conforming to this code displays a HONcode seal on the site. More information about HON and the following Principles, displayed in Table 9.2, can be found at **www.hon.ch**

The fact that a given Web site does not bear the HONcode seal is NOT necessarily an indication of poor quality. The Web is growing so fast and is so diverse that HON (or any other single organization, for that matter) is unlikely ever to review and monitor all sites with possible health care–related content.

Table 9.2. HON code of conduct for medical and health Web sites:
principles (reprinted from Health On the Net Web site).

1. Authority	Any medical or health advice provided and hosted on this site will only be given by medically trained and qualified professionals unless a clear statement is made that a piece of advice offered is from a non-medically qualified individual or organisation.
2. Complementarity	The information provided on this site is designed to support, not replace, the relationship that exists between a patient/site visitor and his/her existing physician.
3. Confidentiality	Confidentiality of data relating to individual patients and visitors to a medical/health Web site, including their identity, is respected by this Web site. The Web site owners undertake to honour or exceed the legal requirements of medical/health information privacy that apply in the country and state where the Web site and mirror sites are located.
4. Attribution	Where appropriate, information contained on this site will be supported by clear references to source data and, where possible, have specific HTML links to that data. The date when a clinical page was last modified will be clearly displayed (e.g. at the bottom of the page).
5. Justifiability	Any claims relating to the benefits/ performance of a specific treatment, commercial product or service will be supported by appropriate, balanced evidence in the manner outlined above in Principle 4.
6. Transparency of authorship	The designers of this Web site will seek to provide information in the clearest possible manner and provide contact addresses for visitors that seek further information or support. The Webmaster will display his/her E-mail address clearly throughout the Web site.

Table 9.2. HON code of conduct for medical and health Web sites: principles (reprinted from Health On the Net Web site).

7. Transparency of sponsorship	Support for this Web site will be clearly identified, including the identities of commercial and non-commercial organisations that have contributed funding, services or material for the site.
8. Honesty in advertising & editorial policy	If advertising is a source of funding it will be clearly stated. A brief description of the advertising policy adopted by the Web site owners will be displayed on the site. Advertising and other promotional material will be presented to viewers in a manner and context that facilitates differentiation between it and the original material created by the institution operating the site.

Citing Information from the Internet

Intellectual property laws apply to all Internet materials including audio, video, graphics, and text. It is necessary to cite Internet sources used in your research and writing just as you cite conventional print-based sources. Gudielines for citing information from the Internet according to American Psychology Association (APA) format are found at **http://www.apa.org/journals/webref.html** and in Modern Language Association (MLA) style at **http://www.mla.org**.

10
The Future Is Now

The role of the Internet in the business world has grown phenomonally over the last ten years. What was seen as "a toy for the computer geek" is now integral to the way we do business. The role of the Internet in health care is poised for the same sort of growth. Several of the health care applications that will be prominent in the next ten years are already being used on the Internet in small or developmental ways. As the role of the Internet develops in health care, these and other applications will gain in popularity and use.

Health Services Over the Internet

Millions of people around the world access health information on the Internet. Health care consumers can be much more knowledgeable about their concerns than ever before. In addition to providing static health information, the Internet offers a variety of interactive health service options.

Health care service providers are slowly beginning to use e-mail to communicate with their clients. One benefit of using e-mail to present your concerns to your provider is that it requires you to be succinct and specific. Another benefit is that it gives the provider an opportunity to prepare or obtain information needed to address your questions prior to any face-to-face meeting. The major issue when communicating with a health care provider by e-mail is confidentiality. Here are some tips to protect yourself:

- Only use your private e-mail account from your home computer. E-mails sent from a company Internet account could be legally archived and/or read by your employer.
- Be careful of the information that you send via e-mail. Due to the way the Internet works, a copy of your message will exist on every computer that is used to deliver your message.
- Verify that the e-mail address you are sending to is actually that of your provider, before you send that sensitive information!
- Confirm how often the provider reads their e-mail messages and who else at the provider's location will have access to your messages.

Encryption tools are available today to protect your messages as they travel over the Internet, but these tools are not generally implemented.

Internet-based video and data transmissions allow health care providers to hold consultations with people who are often in remote geographic areas or unable to travel to the provider. In addition, specialists can provide adjunct consultation services to local health care providers. For example, a heart specialist can view a real-time electrocardiogram of a patient from a thousand miles away and provide expert consultation to the on-site health care provider. Some providers use simple Web-based digital cameras (Webcams) to allow patients to display physical signs and symptoms to the provider without the patient leaving home. Many countries are beginning to invest substantially in telehealth infrastructure and programming.

There are a variety of health service providers who host on-line chat rooms. Many of the chat rooms also have a place to submit questions and the provider, often a physician, will answer them conifdentially. These "on-line office hours" are used by people around the world to gain personal health information. The caution here is to verify the credentials of the person providing the consultation or information. Health Management Organizations (HMOs) and Health Regions often sponsor these types of services for their constituents.

Thousands of other chat rooms dedicated to health are found on the Internet. People can discuss their specific health concerns with others having similar concerns. Many disease or condition-oriented organizations host chat rooms to provide support and practical information for their members.

E-Commerce

The intersection of health and e-commerce has led to a proliferation of on-line sites for purchasing health-related equipment and supplies. A large variety of therapeutic devices, such as light therapy equipment, can be purchased in this way. Many herbal and vitamin products can already be purchased over the Internet. There are several reputable sites offering on-line prescription drug purchase options. The whole area of health e-commerce will see large growth throughout the decade as regulators come to grips with the implications of this trend and implement appropriate policies.

On-line Professional Education

There are many on-line opportunities today to take individual courses for continuing education credit. The growth in the next decade will be in the offering of complete degree programs over the Internet. For example, Athabasca University in Canada currently offers a complete Master of Health Studies degree entirely delivered over the Internet (see **www.athabascau.ca/cnhs**).

E-books

Publishers and bookstores are beginning to develop the processes for publishing and distributing electronic books. This will be an area of rapid growth in the next decade once the mechanisms for copyright and royalties are worked out. An example of an e-book can be found at **http://www.carol-cooper.co.uk/ book/** . This e-book uses simple Web browser technology to present eleven chapters plus a glossary of information about the Internet and other communication technologies. More elaborate tools such as portable hand-held e-book readers are in development.

Conclusion

It is clear that the Internet will greatly affect the practice of health care professionals in every way, from how you find the latest information to how you provide patient care. It is critical that each professional become aware of and proficient in the use of the developing technology and Internet applications, to provide the best possible health care service.

Appendix 1:
Under the Hood

When the earliest cars were built, there was no hood over the engine. You could watch the fan turning and the belts moving and see the steering mechanism in action. As later models were developed, many of these operations were put under the hood and out of your reach. You no longer had to hand-crank the engine to get it started, and you could not see the engine parts in action. Today, you can't even adjust the car's ignition because it is all computerized. The development of the Internet has many parallels to the development of the car. Today when using the Internet, all you have to do is point to an icon and click the mouse button. It has not always been so! This appendix describes some of the earlier Internet tools, and the history of their development.

The Gopher

Any of these information retrieval tools can best be understood as part of an on-going evolutionary process. FTP allowed you to browse through the files of a remote host site. This took a great deal of time, and the results were haphazard and much less than thorough. For success, you had to already know the file name you needed and which computer to try looking on. Archie was an answer to this problem. With an Archie server, you could specify a file name to use to search all FTP sites. The problem then with Archie was that you didn't always know what the contents of the file were simply by looking at the name of a file. *Gopher* was the answer to that problem.

Gopher was developed to help you to know what is in each file. This is accomplished by an administrator at each site that is a designated *Gopher site*. The administrator starts by examining the contents of all files at that Gopher site. Each file is then categorized in one or more ways. By looking at all the categories, the administrator can group files together. Those groupings form Gopher menu pages. Each file in the group is an item on the menu page and has a descriptive title line. Often the menu pages can be arranged in a hierarchical fashion. The administrator then builds links between the menu pages to reflect this hierarchy.

Figure A1.1 is the main Gopher menu page at the Healthline Gopher site. Each item on this page represents a link to a submenu page. For example, when you select the item "General Health Information," you get the menu as illustrated in Figure 6.2.

The first four items are again links to more submenu pages. The other items such as "Asthma" are documents that you can read.

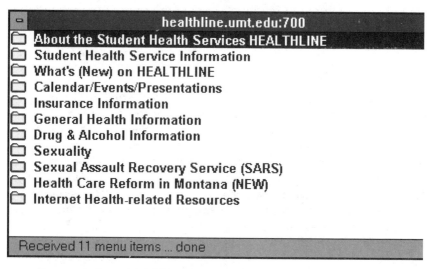

Figure A1.1. Main menu page of HEALTHLINE gopher.

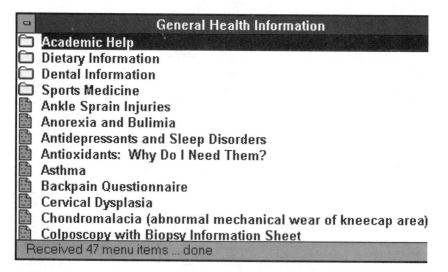

Figure A1.2. Example of submenu Gopher page.

This is only the first screen of the submenu under "General Health Information." There is a total of 47 items on this submenu. You can see the rest by moving down the page.

All Gopher servers are registered with a main Gopher site at the University of Minnesota, the originator of Gopher. Although much folklore exists about the name, the gopher is the mascot of the University of Minnesota, and was chosen as the name by the program originators.

Gopher Searching

You can find information at a Gopher site by personally browsing through many layers of menus until you find what you want. An analogy would be if you were looking for information about *anonymous* in this book, with only the chapter titles and no index available. You would have to make predictions about which chapter you thought that information would be in. Then you would have to skim through the entire chapter to see if the information really was in that chapter. If it wasn't, then you would make another guess and try again. That's how Gopher works. You flip through menu pages selecting items that you think might lead you to where you want to go. If you don't want to go anywhere, Gopher is a terrific way to page through and serendipitously find all kinds of interesting (and sometimes even useful) information on the Internet.

Eventually, people became tired of paging through menus and decided that a better search tool was needed. Using the book analogy, it would be the same as reading through a few chapters and not finding what you want. So you give the book to an assistant with instructions to find the information. That assistant is analogous to the information retrieval system called *Veronica* (yes, to keep Archie company).

Veronica and Jughead Searching

Veronica is a program that searches all gopher sites on a regular basis and takes copies of all the items on all their menu pages. Veronica then indexes the keyword in each menu item. When you do a Veronica search, you search by keyword through all of *gopherspace* (the sum of all Gopher menu items of all Gopher sites in the world). This tool makes finding information at Gopher sites a very simple process. However, if you want to find information from a specific Gopher site, Veronica may not be the right tool for the job.

Jughead was created to search by keyword in the menus and submenus of a specific Gopher site only. Jughead allows you to select the Gopher site and then specify the search terms. Jughead will then search and retrieve information that is located on the Gopher server that you selected.

Wais

Another information retrieval program is *Wais* (Wide Area Information Servers, pronounced wayz). Wais can search any of hundreds of collections of data (called a source) that have been stored as Wais documents. You specify the name of the source and the keywords that you want to search. Wais then searches the sources that you specified. One of the advantages of Wais is that it searches the actual contents of documents, not just the document name. Problems arise with Wais if you don't know what source to specify or if Wais doesn't access the source that you want. Also, because Wais searches for any occurrence of the keyword you specify, if the keyword has more than one contextual meaning, you may get many search items that have no relevance to your real request. If you do not have Windows application software on your computer, Wais is very difficult to use. With Windows-based software, it is much less difficult. Wais is not one of the most popular information retrieval systems, largely because of the limited number of sources and the past difficulty with non-Windows–based access. If the source that you wish to search is available to Wais and you have a Windows-based application, Wais can provide an excellent way to accomplish an in-depth search of Wais documents.

Appendix 2
Health-Related Internet Resources

Profession Specific

Medical Laboratory Technology

International Association of Medical Laboratory Technologists (IAMLT)

Offers conference listings, position papers, employment opportunities, and links
to a variety of specialty-based associations.
World Wide Web:
URL: http://www.iamlt.org/

Medical and Laboratory Sites

This site has extensive links to related sites. A good place to start looking in the
Medical Lab world.
World Wide Web:
URL: http://www.ualberta.ca/~pletendr/medical.html

Listserver

MEDLAB-L
> To join, send mail to **listserv@vm.ucs.ualberta.ca** with **subscribe
> MEDLAB-L <first name> <last name>** in the body of the message.

Nursing

Academic Journal Directory

Contains listings for over 400 professional academic journals related to clinical nursing, nursing education, research, and related healthcare fields. Each listing includes journal name, publisher, frequency of publication, types of manuscripts it reviews, and submission guidelines.
World Wide Web:
URL: http://www.son.utmb.edu/catalog/ajdindex.htm

American Nurses Association

Offers position papers, links to journals, and local associations.
World Wide Web:
URL: http://www.nursingworld.org/

Galaxy Index of Nursing-Related Services on the Internet

Provides extensive links to other nursing-related resources available on the Internet, including Nursing Research, Nursing Theory, and Nursing Specialties. Also includes links to professional, and academic organizations, and student and employment resources.
World Wide Web:
URL: http://health.galaxy.com/

HEALTHWEB: NURSING

Provides information and links related to career information, clinical nursing, education, organizations, research, and other resources.
World Wide Web:
URL: http://www.healthweb.org

Nursesportal.com

This is one of the key places to start looking for nursing information. Formerly Virtualnurse.com, this very large site is searchable, and has information related to education, employment, specialties, chat rooms, and links to other sites.
World Wide Web:
URL: http://www.nursesportal.com

Nursing and the NCLEX

Has links to information about the types of question, scoring, and test plan of the NCLEX. Sample questions from a variety of areas are also available.
World Wide Web:
URL: http://www.ncsbn.org/

NursingNet

Another large searchable nursing portal. Education, employment, links to publications, forums, and chat rooms can all be found here. This is an excellent place to look for nursing resources!
World Wide Web:
URL: http://www.nursingnet.org/

The "Virtual" Nursing Center

Another large nursing information site with links to education, associations, conferences, health topics, and journals.
World Wide Web:
URL: http://www-sci.lib.uci.edu/HSG/Nursing.html

Listservers

CULTURE-AND-NURSING
To join, send mail to **majordomo@itssrvll.ucsf**.edu with **subscribe CULTURE-AND-NURSING** in the body of the message

GradNrse (Graduate Nurses List)
To join, send mail to **LISTSERV@KENTVM.KENT.EDU** with **SUB GradNrse <first-name> <last-name>** in the body of the message.

Ivtherapy-L (IV therapy nursing)
To join, send mail to **majordomo@netcom.com** with **subscribe ivtherapy-L <first-name> <last-name>** in the body of the message.

NURSENET
To join, send mail to **listserv@listserv.utoronto.ca** with **sub nursenet <first-name> <last-name>** in the body of the message.

NURSERES (Nurses Research List)
To join, send mail to **LISTSERV@KENTVM.KENT.EDU** with **SUB NURSERES <first-name> <last-name>** in the body of the message.

NURSE-UK (UK nursing issues)
To join, send mail to **nurse-uk-request@csv.warwick.ac.uk** with **subscribe NURSE-UK <first name> <last name>** in the body of the message.

NRSINGED (Nursing Educators List)
To join, send mail to **listserv@ulkyvm.louisville.edu** with **SUB NRSINGED <first-name> <last-name>** in the body of the message.

NRSING-L (Nursing Informatics List)
>   To join, send mail to **listproc@nic.umass.edu** with **SUB nrsing-l <first-name> <last-name>** in the body of the message.

SCHLRN-L (School nurse list)
>   To join, send mail to **LISTSERV@UBVM.CC.BUFFALO.EDU** with **SUB CHLRN-L <first name> <last name>** in the body of the message.

SNURS-L (For undergraduate nursing students)
>   To join, send mail to **listserv@abvm.cc.buffalo.edu** with **SUB snurse-l <first name> <last name>** in the body of the message.

Newsgroup:

Usenet:
>   newsgroup: **alt.npractitioners** (for nurse practitioners)
>   newsgroup: **sci.med.nursing**
>   newsgroup: **bit.listserv.snurse-l** (for student nurses)

Nutrition

American Dietetics Association

Information, policy papers, employment, and upcoming conferences.
World Wide Web:
URL: http://www.eatright.org/

American Institute of Nutrition

Information about the institute, awards and competitions, publications, and membership information.
World Wide Web:
URL: http://www.faseb.org/ain

Food Science and Technology at Cornell University

Provides links to information about its on-campus and distance education courses.
World Wide Web:
URL: http://aruba.nysaes.cornell.edu/

Occupational Therapy

American Occupational Therapy Association

A good list of links to a variety of occupational therapy associations, information, and resources.
World Wide Web:
URL: http://www.aota.org/

Pharmacy

The "Virtual" Pharmacy Center

Offers links to pharmacy schools, courses, and educational resources.
World Wide Web:
URL: http://www-sci.lib.uci.edu/HSG/Pharmacy.html

Physician Assistants

American Academy of Physician Assistants

Provides links to information about physician assistants, undergraduate and graduate level educational programs, research, resource lists, and job vacancy announcements.
World Wide Web:
URL http://www.aapa.org/

Physiotherapy

American Physical Therapy Association

Offers information related to practice, research, education, news, events, other associations, and products and services. A good place to start.
World Wide Web:
URL: https://www.apta.org/

HealthWeb: Physical Medicine/Physical Therapy

Evaluated resources for the physical medicine community includes links to specific associations and centers, educational tools, and publications. A good beginning site for PTs.
World Wide Web:
URL: http://healthweb.org/browse.cfm?subjectid=74

Physiotherapy Global-Links

An excellent site with journal articles and abstracts, research groups, schools & courses, conference announcements, job opportunities, and links to mailing lists, newsgroups, and other Web sites. Another good place to browse.
World Wide Web:
URL http://ptglobal.net/

Listserver

PHYSIO
> To join, send mail to **mailbase@mailbase.ac.uk** with **subscribe PHYSIO <first name> <last name>** in the body of the message.

Respiratory Therapy

American Association for Respiratory Care

Links to international and national associations education, news, conferences, and services.
World Wide Web:
URL: http://www.aarc.org/

Respiratory Hot-Links

An extensive site providing on-line articles and links to other resources and sites related to specific disorders, employment, education, and publications.
World Wide Web:
URL: http://www.xmission.com/~gastown/herpmed/respi.htm

Newsgroup

Usenet:
> newsgroup: **bit.med.resp-care.world**

Health-Related Topics

Addictions

Canadian Center on Substance Abuse

Offers one of the most up-to-date set of links to information and publications on substance abuse. Also a good source for statistics and publications.
World Wide Web:
URL: http://www.ccsa.ca/

HabitSmart Medical

Offers links to information about addictive behavior, theories of habit endurance and habit change, and tips for effectively managing problematic habitual behavior. Drug and alcohol abuse and adolescent experimentation is well covered. There are several self-administered instruments, articles with suggestions for changing behavior, and a family page with information for parents and kids.
World Wide Web:
URL: http://www.habitsmart.com/

Virtual Clearinghouse on Alcohol, Tobacco, and Other Drugs

This site is a collaboration of a variety of organizations disseminating high-quality information about the nature, extent and consequences of alcohol, tobacco, and other drug use. It is available in English, French, and Spanish. Includes a large selection of full-text documents, calendar of events, and links to other sites.
World Wide Web:
URL: http://www.atod.org/

Web of Addictions

Provides facts sheets on a variety of drugs, in-depth information on specific topics, links to upcoming conferences, other resources, and places to get help with addictions. This site is directed more at the public than health professionals, but is still a good resource.
World Wide Web:
URL: http://www.well.com/user/woa/

Newsgroup

Usenet:
 newsgroup: **alt.recovery**

Listservers

DRUGABUS (related to drug abuse education information and research)
 To join, send mail to **listserv@umab.umd.edu** with **sub drugabus <first name> <last name>** in the body of the message.
Addict-l
 To join, send mail to **listserv@kentvm.kent.edu** with **subscribe addict-l <first name> <last name>** in the body of the message.

Aging

Administration on Aging: Internet and E-mail Resources on Aging

This is THE most extensive listing of resources related to aging, approximately 700! Sometimes referred to as the Post List.
World Wide Web:
URL: http://www.aoa.dhhs.gov/agingsites/default.htm

GoldenAge Net

Offers extensive links to resources related to long-term care and assisted living, commercial sites targeting seniors and their families, government sites, health sites, and a directory of seniors' home pages.
World Wide Web:
URL: http://www.mediasrv.swt.edu/goldenage/intro.htm

Health After 50

The Johns Hopkins Medical Letter is a monthly publication providing medical information and advice for those over 50. Selected articles from each issue are available at this site.
World Wide Web:
URL: http://www.hopkinsafter50.com/

Institute on Aging at the University of Pennsylvania

In addition to links to other resources, this site offers the Turtle Springs Virtual Seniors Community, which provides health information, a newsstand, gazebo chat room, and library. An interesting and colorful site!
World Wide Web:
URL: http://www.med.upenn.edu/~aging/

U.S. Administration on Aging: Directory of Web and Gopher Aging Sites

Links include governmental and nongovernmental agencies, international sites, long-term care topics, mental health concerns including Alzheimer's and related dementias, and libraries and databases.
World Wide Web:
URL: http://www.aoa.dhhs.gov/aoa/webres/craig.htm

The American Association of Retired Persons Guide to Internet Resources Related to Aging

This large searchable site is an excellent place to start looking for information related to aging.
World Wide Web:
URL: http://www.aarp.org/cyber/guide1.htm

AIDS/HIV

AIDS Resource List: Regional, National, and International Sites

This site has many excellent links; however, the choice of background color for the screens makes it difficult to look at for very long.
World Wide Web:
URL: http://www.teleport.com/~celinec/aids.shtml

CDC National Prevention Information Network

Includes current statistics, surveillance reports, general information about prevention and treatment, workplace information, and living with AIDS/HIV, STD, and TB and the connections between them.
World Wide Web:
URL: http://www.cdcnpin.org/

MedWeb: AIDS/HIV

This site only offers links to an extensive list of other resources. You could spend a lot of time browsing this site!
World Wide Web:
URL: http://www.medweb.emory.edu/MedWeb/

National Library of Medicine AIDS Information

Includes AIDSDRUGS database, information services for HIV/AIDS, and an extensive and current bibliography.
World Wide Web:
URL: http://sis.nlm.nih.gov/hiv.cfm

WHO Global Programme on AIDS

Includes information related to this WHO initiative, epidemiology status and trends, women and AIDS, AIDS strategy, research, and links to other sites.
World Wide Web:
URL: http://www.unaids.org/
Gopher:
URL: gopher://gpagopher.who.ch/

WWW Virtual Library: AIDS

A virtual library page with links to sites dealing with the social, political, and medical aspects of AIDS. A good place to begin searching this topic. Some information on sexually transmitted diseases is also included.
World Wide Web:
URL: http://mcb.harvard.edu/BioLinks.html

Yahoo AIDS List

An excellent WWW site providing links to AIDS-related information, resource centers, organizations, and an on-line version of the biweekly AIDS Information Newsletter.
World Wide Web:
URL: http://www.yahoo.com/Health/
Diseases_and_Conditions/AIDS_HIV

Newsgroups

Usenet:
      newsgroup: **clari.tw.health.aids**
      newsgroup: **misc.health.aids**

newsgroup: **sci.med.aids** (moderated)
newsgroup: HIV.AIDS.ARC
newsgroup: HIV.AIDS.LAW
newsgroup: HIV.AIDS.SPIRITUAL
newsgroup: HIV.AIDS.WOMEN

Allergies and Asthma

Allergy, Asthma & Immunology Online

This site is maintained by the American College of Allergy, Asthma, and Immunology. It includes information for patients, physicians, news about allergy and asthma, and links to other Web sites. This site is searchable.
World Wide Web:
URL: http://allergy.mcg.edu/

Allergy and Asthma Web Page

This started as the **misc.kids** Allergy and Asthma FAQ, so it is geared to the public, especially parents. Not an elegant site, but good information on resources, book reviews, and an extensive collection of recipes.
World Wide Web:
URL: http://www.cs.unc.edu/~kupstas/FAQ.html

Allergy Clean Environments

Offers links to products and services for allergic individuals.
World Wide Web:
URL: http://www.w2.com:80/allergy.html

American Academy of Allergy, Asthma, and Immunology

Provides general information, calendar of events, related organizations, and agencies and scientific information resources.
World Wide Web:
URL: http://www.aaaai.org/

Food Allergy Network

An excellent site for those with food allergies. Includes information, product alerts and updates, and a newsletter that includes allergy-free recipes and answers to diet dilemmas.
World Wide Web:
URL: http://www.foodallergy.org/

Latex Allergy Home Page

Includes advice from your allergist, a link to a management protocol, and a link to a support organization.
World Wide Web:
URL: http://allergy.mcg.edu/physicians/ltxhome.html

National Institute of Allergy and Infectious Diseases

Offers information about a wide variety of allergies and infectious diseases.
World Wide Web:
URL: http://www.niaid.nih.gov/

Newsgroups

Usenet:
>   newsgroup: **alt.med.allergy**
>   newsgroup: **alt.support.asthma**

Alternative Medicine

Alternative Medicine Home Page

Offers information on unconventional, unorthodox, unproven, alternative, complementary, innovative, integrative therapies, including databases, mailing lists and newsgroups, and numerous links to related sites.
World Wide Web:
URL: http://www.pitt.edu/~cbw/altm.html

National Center for Complementary and Alternative Medicine

The National Center for Complementary and Alternative Medicine (NCCAM) at the National Institutes of Health (NIH) conducts and supports basic and applied research and training and disseminates information on complementary and alternative medicine to practitioners and the public. The site includes fact sheets, databases, and clinical trial opportunities.
World Wide Web:
URL: http://nccam.nih.gov/

Yahoo Health: Alternative Medicine

Links to networks, research, journals, and organizations related to alternative and complementary therapies.
World Wide Web:
URL: http://dir.yahoo.com/Health/Alternative_Medicine/

Newsgroups

Usenet:
>   newsgroup: **misc.health.alternative**
>   newsgroup: **alt.health.ayurveda**
>   newsgroup: **soc.religion.shamanism**

Listservers

ALTMED-RES (Alternative medicine research)
>   To join, send mail to **majordomo@virginia.edu** with **subscribe ALTMED-RES <first name> <last name>** in the body of the message.

AROMA-TRIALS (Related to aromatherapy)
>   To join, send mail to **mailbase@mailbase.ac.uk** with **subscribe AROMA-TRIALS <first name> <last name>** in the body of the message.

Alzheimer's Disease

Alzheimer's Disease Center

Contains links to resources for both family and professional caregivers. Also contains several links to neuropathology resources.
World Wide Web:
URL: http://206.119.4.214/alzheimer/

Alzheimer's Disease Education and Referral Center

In addition to offering information, research, and publications related to Alzheimer's disease, there is also the ability to submit questions to be answered by specialists.
World Wide Web:
URL: http://www.alzheimers.org/

Alzheimer Web

Provides links to news items, research, articles, conferences, and associations worldwide.
World Wide Web:
URL: http://www.alzweb.org

The Alzheimer Page

The Web page for the Alzheimer mailing list and its digest, Alzheimer-digest. Contains subscription information, searchable archives, and links to related sites.
World Wide Web:
URL: http://www.biostat.wustl.edu/alzheimer/

Listserver

ALZHEIMER
To join, send mail to MARJORDOMO@WUBOIS.WUSTL.EDU with **subscribe ALZHEIMER <first name> <last name>** in the body of the message.

Arthritis

American College of Rheumatology Home Page

While largely offering services to its members, this site also offers excellent patient information, an on-line version of "ACR News," and upcoming meetings.
World Wide Web:
URL: http://www.rheumatology.org/index.asp

Arthritis Foundation
A good place to start. Includes news and facts, a list of local offices, research resources and awards, information about "Arthritis Today," advocacy resources, information for health professional, and a section on juvenile arthritis.
World Wide Web:
URL: http://www.arthritis.org/

Arthritis National Research Foundation
This site is focused on arthritis research, listing grants, conferences, and other related information.
World Wide Web:
URL: http://www.curearthritis.org/

HealthWeb: Rheumatology

Links to consumer and patient information, clinical trials, reference documents for health professionals related to a variety of rheumatology topics including carpal tunnel syndrome, fibromyalgia, and chronic fatigue syndrome.
World Wide Web:
URL: http://www.medlib.iupui.edu/hw/rheuma/disease.html

Learning to Live with Arthritis

Management strategies for the person with arthritis. Practical information related to a variety of topics such as diet, exercises, fatigue, pregnancy, and travel.
World Wide Web:
URL: http://www.orthop.washington.edu/Bone%20and%20Joint%20Sources/xxxxxxxz1_1.html (yes, 8 exes!)

National Institute of Arthritis and Musculoskeletal and Skin Diseases

Part of the National Institutes for Health, this site provides fact sheets, statistics, bibliographies, consensus conference reports, information on clinical trials, grants, and news and events.
World Wide Web:
URL: http://www.nih.gov/niams

Newsgroups

Usenet:
>   newsgroup: **alt.support.arthritis**
>   newsgroup: **misc.health.arthritis**

Attention Deficit Disorder

ADDNet

Full-text articles relating to interventions, particularly for educators.
Gopher:
URL: gopher://moe.coe.uga.edu:70/11/1TN%3A%Interactive%20Teaching%20Network%20of%20UGA/A N

National Attention Deficit Disorder Association (ADDA)

This is a good starting point. Information related to parents, adults, legal concerns, employee assistance programs, medications, adult support groups, and an on-line journal for adults. Excellent links to other resources.
World Wide Web:
URL: http://www.add.org/Y

Newsgroup

Newsgroup: **alt.support.attn-deficit**

Breast Cancer

American Cancer Society's Breast Cancer Resource Center

Designed to provide information to patients and their families. Includes breast self-exam (BSE) teaching, treatment options, and extensive links to other on-line information. The site to start with in searching for information about breast cancer!
World Wide Web:
URL: http://www3.cancer.org/cancerinfo/load_cont.asp?ct=5

CancerNet: A Service of the National Cancer Institute: Breast Cancer

This is a comprehensive site with links and information about statistics, clinical trials, risk factors, prevention, complementary and alternative therapies, and support and resources. There is an excellent section called "What you need to know" that would be a great starting place for learning about breast cancer.
World Wide Web:
URL http://cancernet.nci.nih.gov/cancer_types/breast_cancer.shtml

Community Breast Health Project

The mission of the Community Breast Health Project is to improve the lives of people touched by breast cancer by acting as a clearinghouse for information and support, providing volunteer opportunities for breast cancer survivors and friends dedicated to helping others with the disease, and serving as an educational resource and a community center for all who are concerned about breast cancer and breast health. The Community Breast Health Project is grass-roots, patient-driven, and committed to providing services free of charge.
World Wide Web:
URL http://www-med.stanford.edu/CBHP/

National Alliance of Breast Cancer Organizations

Over 400 organizations are included in this alliance. The site offers information about new developments, conferences and workshops, lay and professional resources, support groups, and clinical trials.
World Wide Web:
URL: http://www.nabco.org/info/index.html

National Breast Cancer Coalition Web Site

This is the Web site for a grass-roots coalition formed to eradicate breast cancer through action and advocacy. Find information about current programs and new campaigns at this site.
World Wide Web:
URL: http://www.natlbcc.org/

Oncolink

Provides information about the nature of cancer, breast self-exam and mammography guidelines, psychological issues, and risk factors.
World Wide Web:
URL: http://cancer.med.upenn.edu/disease/breast/

Cancer

American Cancer Society

This site provides links to local, national, and international organizations, local resources, information about types of cancer, and treatment options. It includes a tool called "CancerProfiler" designed to help determine the best treatment options for someone diagnosed with cancer. It is also the home of the Cancer Survivors Network, for cancer survivors and caregivers.
World Wide Web:
URL http://www.cancer.org/

CancerNet

This is an extensive site offering links to information about various types of cancer, treatment options, clinical trials, risk factors, prevention, testing, and support and resources. This site also hosts the CancerLit searchable database of relevant articles. Physician Data Query (PDQ) contains peer-reviewed summaries on cancer treatment, screening, prevention, genetics, and supportive

care, and a registry of open and closed cancer clinical trials from around the world.
World Wide Web:
URL: http://cnetdb.nci.nih.gov/index.html

National Cancer Institute

Offers extensive links to cancer information, resources for scientists, partnerships, including advocacy groups, and the "Cancer Information Service," which provides information about new developments related to cancer.
World Wide Web:
URL: http://www.nci.nih.gov/

OncoLink

Contains links to disease oriented menus, specialty oriented menus, psychological support, support groups, cancer organizations, spirituality, clinical trials, and other cancer resources.
World Wide Web:
URL: http://cancer.med.upenn.edu/

Talaria: The Hypermedia Assistant for Cancer Pain Management

Provides a hypermedia implementation of the Clinical Practice Guideline on the Management of Cancer Pain (U.S. Dept. of Health). Includes assessment guidelines, pharmacologic and nonpharmocologic management, non-pharma-cologic interventions, a discussion of procedure-related pain in children and adults, and a description of how to monitor the quality of pain management.
World Wide Web:
URL: http://www.talaria.org

Newsgroups

Usenet:
>   newsgroup: **alt.support.cancer**
>   newsgroup: **sci.med.diseases.cancer**

Listserver

CANCER-L (Public list for cancer-related issues)
>   To join, send mail to **listserv@wvnvm.wvnet.edu** with **subscribe CANCER-L <first name> <last name>** in the body of the message.

Celiac Disease

Celiac Discussion List Archives

As the title says, this archive contains on-line articles related to celiac disease, gluten-free diet information, links to the discussion list, and to other resources.
World Wide Web:
URL: http://www.fastlane.net/homepages/thodge/archive.htm

National Institute of Diabetes and Digestive and Kidney Diseases (NIDDK): Celiac Disease

This site offers information about celiac disease, its diagnosis, and treatment.
World Wide Web:
URL: http://www.niddk.nih.gov/health/digest/pubs/celiac/#10

WWWebguides: Information for Gluten-free and Wheat-free Diets

Offers full text articles, recipes, support group information, and commercial product information.
World Wide Web:
URL: http://www.wwwebguides.com/nutrition/diets/glutenfree

Listserver

CELIAC
    To join, send mail to **listserv@sjuvm.st.johns.edu** with **sub CELIAC <first name> <last name>** in the body of the message.

Children's Health

Harriet Lane Links (formerly Pediatric Points of Interest)

Although it sounds medically oriented, this searchable site has good information for both the public and health care professionals.
World Wide Web:
URL: http://www.med.jhu.edu/peds/neonatology/poi.html

Health Oasis: Children's Health Center

Health Oasis is a function of the Mayo Clinic. It offers news briefs, full text reference articles, and links to sites designed for children.
World Wide Web:
URL http://www.mayohealth.org/mayo/common/htm/pregpg.htm

KidsHealth

Excellent information and resources for kids, parents, and professionals related to a variety of topics including growth and development, nutrition, surgery, immunizations, lab tests, and recipes.
World Wide Web:
URL: http://KidsHealth.org/

Newsgroup

Usenet:
>   newsgroup: **misc.kids.health**

Listserver

PEDIATRIC-PAIN
>   To join, send mail to **mailserv@ac.dal.ca** with **subscribe PEDIATRIC-PAIN <first name> <last name>** in the body of the message.

Chronic Fatigue Syndrome

The Chronic Fatigue and Immune Dysfunction Syndrome Association of America

This is a well-maintained site offering information on CFIDS, pediatric CFIDS, educational resources, an on-line newsletter, and good links to other resources.
World Wide Web:
URL: http://www.cfids.org/

The Facts About Chronic Fatigue Syndrome

This CDC site provides on-line information about possible causes, diagnosis, clinical aspects, and demographics of CFS. There is a large references and publications section with some full text articles.
World Wide Web:
URL: http://www.cdc.gov/ncidod/diseases/cfs/index.htm

Newsgroup

Usenet:
  newsgroup: **alt.med.cfs**

Communicable Diseases

Centers for Disease Control

Provides extensive, searchable information and statistics related to prevention, incidence, and immunization guidelines related to both common and unusual diseases. Includes guidelines for travelers.
World Wide Web:
URL: http://www.cdc.gov/

Infectious Disease Weblink: Infectious Disease Specialty Supersite

This is a large, searchable site offering links to new developments, practice guidelines, lectures, conference highlights, other resources, and clinical images.
World Wide Web:
URL: http://pages.prodigy.net/pdeziel/

Immunization Action Coalition

Offers vaccine information statements, free print material in 17 languages, links to national resources, and strategies to improve immunization rates.
World Wide Web:
URL: http://www.immunize.org/

WWW Travel Health Information

Provides links to information about diseases, immunization, environmental hazards, travel warnings, and preventative measures.
World Wide Web:
URL: http://www.intmed.mcw.edu/travel.html

Community Health

International Network for Interfaith Health Practices

Offers information, model practices, and other health resources related to the interaction of faith and health. Particular resources for Parish nurses
World Wide Web:
URL: http://www.interaccess.com/ihpnet Y

The "Virtual" Public Health Center

Links to public health schools, courses and education resources, demography, and population databases. Also extensive information related to a variety of public health topics. A good place to start searching this topic.
World Wide Web:
URL: http://www-sci.lib.uci.edu/HSG/PHealth.html Y

WHO Collaborating Center for Research on Healthy Cities

Links to current and archived newsletters, groups throughout the world, and on-line information about the project.
World Wide Web:
URL: http://www.rulimburg.nl/~who-city/www.html Y

Listservers

Community Mobilization/development
> To join, send mail to **listserv@zeus.med.uottawa.ca** with **subscribe community_mobilization/development <first name> <last name>** in the body of the message
General Community Health Issues
> To join, send mail to **listserv@zeus.med.uottawa.ca** with **subscribe general_community_health_issues <first name> <last name>** in the body of the message.
International Network for Interfaith Health Practices (formerly Parish Nurses)
> To join, send mail to **IHP-NET-REQUEST@synasoft**.com with **subscribe <first name> <last name>** in the body of the message.
PUBLIC-HEALTH
> To join, send mail to **mailbase@mailbase.ac.uk** with **subscribe PUBLIC-HEALTH <first name> <last name>** in the body of the message.
Rural-Care
> To join, send mail to **majordomo@avocado.pc.helsinki.fi with subscribe Rural-Care <first name> <last name>** in the body of the message.
RURALNET-L

To join, send mail to **listserv@musom01.mu.wvnet.edu** with **subscribe RURALNET-L \<first name\> \<last name\>** in the body of the message.

Cystic Fibrosis

Cystic Fibrosis Foundation

Provides information, news updates, clinical trial information, publications (some on-line), membership information, and links to other resources.
World Wide Web:
URL: http://www.cff.org/

Cystic Fibrosis Resource Page

This page is intended to be an exhaustive guide to all web pages, mailing lists, FAQs, and newsgroups related to cystic fibrosis. It certainly lives up to its claims.
World Wide Web:
URL: http://vmsb.csd.mu.edu/~5418lukasr/cystic.html

Listserver

Cystic-L
   To join, send mail to **listserv@Yalevm.cis.Yale.edu** with **subscribe cystic-l \<first name\> \<last name\>** in the body of the message.

Depression

Internet Depression Resources

Also offers good links to organizations, archives of several newsgroups and their respective FAQs, direct links to subscribe to a variety of mailing lists, and information on what to say and what not to say to a depressed person.
World Wide Web:
URL: http://stripe.colorado.edu/~judy/depression/

MentalHealth Net: Depression

This is the place to start looking for information related to depression. Offers information for the public and health professionals, on-line articles, drug

information, support group locations, assessment instruments, and treatment guidelines.
World Wide Web:
URL: http://depression.mentalhelp.net/

Newsgroups

Usenet:
> newsgroup: **alt.psychology.help**
> newsgroup: **alt.support.depression**
> newsgroup: **alt.support.depression.manic**
> newsgroup: **alt.support.depression.seasonal**
> newsgroup: **alt.support.phobias**
> newsgroup: **sci.psychology**
> newsgroup: **sci.med**
> newsgroup: **sci.med.psycobiology**

Diabetes and Other Endocrine Disorders

Children with Diabetes

An on-line resource for children and parents includes general information, a chat room, food and diet information, products, and listings of other resources including camps.
World Wide Web:
URL: http://www.castleweb.com/diabetes/index.html

Diabetes Associations' Home Pages

Provide information about the services offered by the various associations.
American Diabetes Association
World Wide Web:
URL: http://www.diabetes.org
British Diabetic Association
World Wide Web:
URL: http://www.pavilion.co.uk/diabetic/
Canadian Diabetes Association
World Wide Web:
URL: http://www.diabetes.ca
Juvenile Diabetes Foundation
World Wide Web:
URL: http://www.jdf.org/

Diabetes Research International Network

The goal of this site is to make scientific research understandable to those with diabetes. There is information for both the public and health professionals.
World Wide Web:
URL: http://www.drinet.org/html/the_diabetes_research_institut.htm

National Institute of Diabetes & Digestive and Kidney Diseases

Provides links to diabetes statistics, control and complications trials, organizations, and information about diabetic eye disease, insulin-dependent and non–insulin dependent diabetes.
World Wide Web:
URL: http://www.niddk.nih.gov/

Newsgroups

Usenet:
> newsgroup: **misc.health.diabetes**
> newsgroup: **alt.support.diabetes.kids**

Listserver

DIABETES (International research project on diabetes)
> To join, send mail to **listserv@irlearn.ucd.ie** with **subscribe DIABETES <first name> <last name>** in the body of the message.

Digestive Diseases

National Institute of Diabetes and Digestive and Kidney Diseases

Provides links to diabetes statistics, control and complications trials, organizations, and information about diabetic eye disease, insulin-dependent and non–insulin-dependent diabetes. Also lists voluntary and private organizations involved in digestive diseases–related activities, including provision of educational materials.
World Wide Web:
URL: http://www.niddk.nih.gov/

Newsgroup

Usenet:
> newsgroup: **alt.support.crohns-colitis**

Disabilities

ABLEDATA: The National Database of Assistive Technology Information

An extensive, searchable database listing information on assistive technology available both commercially and noncommercially. It offers fact sheets and its own "top ten" searches.
World Wide Web:
URL: http://www.abledata.com

CODI: Cornucopia of Disability Information

A well-maintained repository for disability-related information of all types.
World Wide Web:
URL: http://codi.buffalo.edu/

Communication Disorders and Sciences

Outlines the Internet resources available on communication disorders.
World Wide Web:
URL: http://www.mankato.msus.edu/dept/comdis/kuster2/welcome.html

DISABILITY Resources on the Internet

This site is very extensive and searchable. You'll find everything you're looking for somewhere on this site! This site has links to a organizations, newsletters, and articles related to a variety of disabilities.
World Wide Web:
URL: http://www.eskimo.com/~jlubin/disabled.html

Dyslexia

An excellent place to start looking for resources related to dyslexia. This page has numerous links to other sites, information related to education, support, and other organizations and associations.
World Wide Web:
URL: http://www.dyslexia.uk.com/

Newsgroups

Usenet:
    newsgroup: **misc.handicap**
    newsgroup: **alt.support.dev-delays**

newsgroup: **alt.support.cerebral-palsy**
newsgroup: **alt.support.spina-bifida**

Listserver

bit.listserv.autism
> Children with special health care needs. To join, send mail to **listserv@nervm.nerdc.ufl.edu** with **subscribe cshcn <first name> <last name>** in the body of the message.

Down Syndrome

Down Syndrome WWW Page

Offers links to contributed articles, a medical checklist, worldwide organizations, inclusion and educational resources, parent matching and support groups, conferences, and toy catalogues.
World Wide Web:
URL: http://www.nas.com/downsyn/

Parents Helping Parents

Links to LINCS, a searchable on-line human services directory addressing the needs of children and adults with almost any need for specialized care or services. For those without WWW access, there is an FTP site.
World Wide Web:
URL: http://www.php.com

Listserver

bit.listserv.down-syn
> Children with Down Syndrome. To join, send mail to **listserv@vm1. nodak.edu** with **subscribe down-syn <first name> <last name>** in the body of the message.

Eating Disorders

Internet Mental Health: Anorexia Nervosa: Research Re: Treatment

Full-text articles about current research related to treatment of eating disorders.
World Wide Web:
URL: http://www.mentalhealth.com/dis-rs/frs-et01.html

Mental Health Net: Eating Disorders

Although this site is aimed at the public, there is good information for health professionals also. There are links to a wide variety of resources and support groups, information about recognition, and treatment.
World Wide Web:
URL http://eatingdisorders.mentalhelp.net/

Newsgroup

Usenet:
   newsgroup: **alt.support.eating-disord**

Emergency Medical Services (EMS)

Emergency Nursing World

A large site with links of interest to all EMS practitioners. Includes tips and tricks, pediatric hints, discharge instructions, links to other sites, mailing lists, and newsgroups.
World Wide Web:
URL: http://ENW.org/

Listservers

EMED-L
   Hospital-based emergency medical practitioners. To join, send mail to **listserv@itssrv1.ucsf.edu** with **sub EMED-L <first name> <last name>** in the body of the message.
INJURY-L
   To join, send mail to **listserv@wvnvm.wvnet.edu** with **sub injury-l <first name> <last name>** in the body of the message.

Newsgroups

Usenet:
   newsgroup: **misc.emergency.services**
   newsgroup: **misc.ems**

Endometriosis

Listserver

WITSENDO
> To join, send mail to **listserv@dartcms1.dartmouth.edu** with **sub WITSENDO <first name> <last name>** in the body of the message.

Epilepsy

Epilepsy Foundation

Offers extensive links to other resources, support groups and organizations, information, medications, discussion groups, and mailing lists.
World Wide Web:
URL: http://www.efa.org/

Listservers

Epilepsy-List (for persons living with epilepsy and their families)
> To join, send mail to **listserv@calvin.dgbt.doc.ca** with **subscribe epilepsy-list <first name> <last name>** in the body of the message.

Epilepsy-Pro (for professionals)
> To join, send mail to **listserv@calvin.dgbt.doc.ca** with **subscribe epilepsy-pro <first name> <last name>** in the body of the message.

Newsgroup

Usenet:
> newsgroup: **alt.support.epilepsy**

Ethics

National Reference Center for Bioethics Literature

The National Reference Center for Bioethics Literature (NRCBL) is a specialized collection of books, journals, newspaper articles, legal materials, regulations, codes, government publications, and other relevant documents

concerned with issues in biomedical and professional ethics. Also includes extensive links to other related sites.
World Wide Web:
URL: http://www.georgetown.edu/research/nrcbl/

Listserver

BIOMED-L (related to biomedical ethics)
>   To join, send mail to **listserv@VM1.NODAK.Edu** with **subscribe BIOMED-L <first name> <last name>** in the body of the message.

Evidence-Based Practice

Center for Evidence-based Medicine

Includes a "toolbox," teaching archives, and information about the center and its publications.
World Wide Web:
URL: http://cebm.jr2.ox.ac.uk/

Cochrane Collaboration

This site focuses on preparing, maintaining, and promoting the accessibility of systematic reviews of the effects of health care interventions. There is general information, guidelines, manuals, software, and links to Cochrane groups and country sites.
World Wide Web:
URL: http://www.cochrane.org/

Fibromyalgia

National Fibromyalgia Research Association

Offers links to diagnostic criteria, exercise guidelines, and information resources.
World Wide Web:
URL: http://www.teleport.com/~nfra/

A Physician's Guide to Fibromyalgia Syndrome

Although directed at physicians, there is good information for other health care professionals, including etiology, diagnosis, treatment, and a table of useful drugs.
World Wide Web:
URL: http://www.hsc.missouri.edu/fibro/fm-md.html

Newsgroup

Usenet:
newsgroup: **alt.med.fibromyalgia**

Listserver

FIROM-L
To join, send mail to **listserv@vmd.cso.uiuc.edu** with **sub FIROM-L** **<first name> <last name>** in the body of the message.

Gerontology

The Gerontological Society of America

Extensive links to resources covering all aspects of gerontology, including conferences, grants, and information for the public and health professionals.
World Wide Web:
URL: http://www.geron.org/

Listservers

Fall prevention in the elderly
To join, send mail to **listserv@zeus.med.uottawa.ca** with **subscribe** **fall_prevention_in_the_elderly <first name> <last name>** in the body of the message.
GERINET
To join, send mail to **listserv@ubvm.cc.buffalo.edu-bit.listserv.** **GERINET** with **subscribe GERINET <first name> <last name>** in the body of the message.

Grief

Listserver

grief-chat

> To join, send mail to **majordomo@falcon**.ic.net with **subscribe grief-chat <first name> <last name>** in the body of the message. (There are many specialized groups at this site. This list will help you to connect to a suitable group.)

Newsgroup

Usenet:

> newsgroup: **alt.support.grief**
> newsgroup: **soc.support.pregnancy.loss**

Headache

American Council for Headache Education (ACHE)

This site is dedicated to advancing the treatment and management of headache and to raising the public awareness of headache as a valid, biologically based illness. There are many links to information, resources, and support groups.
World Wide Web:
URL: http://www.achenet.org/

Migraine Resource Center

Offers articles related to triggers, symptoms, treatment programs, diagnostic screening, and latest news.
World Wide Web:
URL: http://www.migrainehelp.com

National Headache Foundation

This site offers information on a variety of headache conditions and treatments, clinical trials, and professional programs.
World Wide Web:
URL: http://www.headaches.org/

Listserver

headache
> To join, send mail to **listserv@shsu.edu** with **subscribe headache <first name> <last name>** in the body of the message.

Newsgroup

Usenet:
> newsgroup: **alt.support.headaches.migraine**

Health

Hardin Meta Directory of Internet Health Sources

This directory contains extensive links to sites directed at both the public and health care professionals related to a variety of topics noted by medical specialty.
World Wide Web:
URL: http://www.lib.uiowa.edu/hardin/md/

Health-related World-Wide Web server

Offers links to an extensive variety of other WWW sites related to health.
World Wide Web:
URL: http://www.who.int/m/healthtopics-a-z/en/index.html

HealthWeb

Provides "organized access to evaluated, noncommercial" Internet resources. A key to this site is that the resources included are evaluated, so standards have been applied to the offerings. There is an extensive listing of topics.
World Wide Web:
URL: http://healthweb.org/index.cfm

Internet Health Newsgroups and Listserver Groups

Provides links to a large variety of newsgroups and listserver groups arranged by health topic. This is a good place to check for new groups that are not found in this catalogue.
World Wide Web:
URL: http://www.ihr.com/newsgrp.html

Magellan: Health and Medicine

Extensive links to a large variety of health resources such as conditions and diseases, personal fitness, personal care, services, and resources. Another excellent place to start browsing. This is a searchable site.
World Wide Web:
URL: http://magellan.excite.com/health/

National Institutes of Health

Offers information on a variety of health topics and also clinical information.
World Wide Web:
URL: http://www.nih.gov

World Health Organization

Includes information about major programs, World Health Report, Weekly Epidemiological Record, WHO's Statistical Information System, World Health Day, public information, newsletters, and international travel requirements and advice.
World Wide Web:
URL: http://www.who.org

Yahoo: Health

Probably the best place to start looking for health-related information. Examples of links include diseases and conditions, education, fitness, general health, health administration, mental health, reproductive health, sexuality, and workplace health. This site is searchable.
World Wide Web:
URL: http://www.yahoo.com/health/

Newsgroup

Usenet:
> newsgroup: **clari.tw.health**

Listservers

HEALTH-L (related to health research)
> To join, send mail to **listserv@irlearn.ucd.ie** with **subscribe HEALTH-L <first name> <last name>** in the body of the message.

HealthNet Listserv
> To join, send mail to **listserv@calvin.dgbt.doc.ca** with **subscribe healthnet <first name><last name>** in the body of the message.

Health Promotion

Health Promotion

Provides submenus that provide information at a lay level to assist individuals to plan and carry out health promotion activities. Submenus relate to back and neck care, body image, breast self-exam, eye care, fast food calorie counter, health promotion suggested timetable, massage, relationships, and testicular self-exam.
World Wide Web:
URL: http://www.uiuc.edu/departments/mckinley/health-info/hlthpro/
hlthpro.html

National Center for Chronic Disease Prevention and Health Promotion: Chronic Disease Prevention

This site provides information about chronic, and preventable diseases and conditions, risk behaviors, surveillance, comprehensive approaches, and

programs designed for specific populations, including maternal and infant health. There is also a large selection of related links.
World Wide Web:
URL http://www.cdc.gov/nccdphp/

Listservers

Behaviour Change Strategies
> To join, send mail to **listserv@zeus.med.uottawa.ca** with **subscribe behavioural_change_strategies <first name> <last name>** in the body of the message.

FIT-L
> To join, send mail to **listserv@etsuadm.etsu.edu** with **sub fit-l <first name> <last name>** in the body of the message.

Newsgroups

Usenet:
> newsgroup: **misc.fitness**
> newsgroup: **su.org.hpp-aerobics**

Heart Health

American Heart Association

Offers on-line articles including "Heart & Stroke A to Z Guide," risk assessment, lists of local resources, and information for health professionals.
World Wide Web:
URL: http://www.americanheart.org/

Arnot Ogden Medical Center: Heart Health

This is an excellent resource for patient teaching materials. There are extensive on-line articles written for the lay person related to all aspects of cardiovascular disease, prevention, surgery, and rehabilitation. Searchable.
World Wide Web:
URL: http://www.aomc.org/HOD2/general/heart-Contents.html

National Heart, Lung, and Blood Institute

This site has excellent health information, scientific resources, clinical guidelines, and public interest news.
World Wide Web:
URL: http://www.nhlbi.nih.gov/index.htm

Home Health

Homecare Online: National Association for Home Care

Offers consumer information, lists of associations, vendor lists, an on-line version of *Caring* magazine, including archives and a listing of upcoming meetings.
World Wide Web:
URL: http://www.nahc.org

Listservers

hcarenurse
> To join, send mail to **majordomo@po.cwru.edu** with **subscribe hcarenurse <your e-mail address>** in the body of the message.

homehlth
> To join, send mail to **listserv@usa.net** with **subscribe homehlth <first-name> <last-name>** in the body of the message.

HOSPICE
> To join, send mail to **majordomo@po.cwru.edu** with **subscribe hospice <your e-mail address>** in the body of the message.

Hospitals

Hospitals on the World Wide Web

Has links to a variety of hospitals around the world. The information provided by the various hospitals is not consistent, but may include department information, site plans, and telephone listings.
World Wide Web:
URL: http://neuro-www.mgh.harvard.edu/hospitalweb.shtml

Immune System Disorders

Listserver

IMMUNE
> To join, send mail message **to IMMUNE-REQUEST@WEBER. UCSD.EDU** with **subscribe IMMUNE <first name> <last name>** in the body of the message.

Informatics

AMIA: Nursing Informatics Working Group

Provides information on current activities, education in nursing informatics, upcoming conferences, and links to related sites.
World Wide Web:
URL: http://www.amia-niwg.org/

COACH: Canada's Health Informatics Association

General information, publications, and conference announcements are found here. Also links to other resources.
World Wide Web:
URL: http://www.coachorg.com/

Duke Medical Informatics

Provides links to other health and medical informatics links worldwide.
World Wide Web:
URL: http://dmi-www.mc.duke.edu/

St. F.X.U. Nursing Informatics

This site offers extensive links to health care informatics sites worldwide. Definitely the place to start searching this topic. Also excellent links to general nursing and health care sites.
World Wide Web:
URL: http://juliet.stfx.ca/people/fac/rmackinn/nursei.html

Newsgroup

Usenet:
  newsgroup: **sci.med.informatics**

Listservers

CPRI-L (related to telecommunications in health care)
  To join, send mail to **listserv@ukanaix.cc.ukans.edu** with **subscribe CPRI-L <first name> <last name>** in the body of the message.
MEDINF-L
  To join, send mail to **listserv@vm.gmd.de** with **subscribe MEDINFO-L <first name> <last name>** in the body of the message.
Nursing Informatics
  To join, send mail to **listproc@lists.umass.edu** with **subscribe nrsing-l <first name> <last name>** in the body of the message.

Job Search

MedSearch America

Provided by a commercial service; allows you to post your resume on-line, search jobs, and search resumes. Also includes information about health care industry resources, career articles, and outlook.
World Wide Web:
URL: http://www.medsearch.com

Kidney and Urologic Disorders

The International Society for Peritoneal Dialysis

Information is available in English, French, Italian, and Spanish. Includes meeting/conference announcements, recommendations for training, recommendations for treatment of peritonitis, a page for nurses, nutritionists, and social workers, and a patient's page.
World Wide Web:
URL: http://www.ispd.org/

National Institute of Diabetes, Digestive and Kidney Disease

Information about various diseases for the public, research information, facts, and statistics for health care professionals.
World Wide Web:
URL: http://www.niddk.nih.gov/

Lupus

Lupus Foundation of America

Offers a detailed FAQ, current information, research library, lists of support groups, and agencies and information related to causes, symptoms, testing, and treatment.
World Wide Web:
URL: http://www.lupus.org/lupus/

Menopause

A Friend Indeed

Provides menopause information and articles and subscription information for the newsletter "A Friend Indeed."
World Wide Web:
URL: http://www.pangea.ca/~afi/

The North American Menopause Society,

This is an excellent site to begin searching this topic. information related to consumer and professional education, conference announcements, and consensus statements.
World Wide Web:
URL: http://www.menopause.org/

Newsgroup

Usenet:
newsgroup: **alt.support.menopause**

Men's Health

American Prostate Society

On this comprehensive site, you will find general information about prostate cancer and prostatitis, and back issues of the society newsletter.
World Wide Web:
URL: http://www.ameripros.org/

Men's Health: Medbroadcast.com

Information on a wide variety of health issues including male menopause, erectile dysfunction, vasectomy, and fatherhood.
World Wide Web:
URL: http://www.medbroadcast.com/health_topics/mens_health/

Mental Health

American Psychological Association

Information related to associations and organizations, DSM criteria, journals, mailing lists, and newsgroups with specific interests. Searchable by topic.
World Wide Web:
URL: http://www.apa.org/

National Institutes of Mental Health

Information related to grants and contracts, publications, on-line education programs, and consensus conference proceedings. For both the public and health care professionals.
World Wide Web:
URL: http://www.nimh.nih.gov

Seasonal Light/Seasonal Affective Disorder Home Page

Provides a list of print resources about SAD, organizations, and information about light sources.
World Wide Web:
URL: http://www.geocities.com/HotSprings/7061/sadhome.html

Yahoo Internet Mental Health Resources

Provides links to information on a variety or medical and mental health topics.
World Wide Web:
URL: http://www.yahoo.com/Health/Mental_Health/

Listserver

PSYCHOPHYSIOLOGY
> To join, send mail to **MAILBASE@MAILBASE.AC.UK** with **JOIN CLINICAL-PSYCHOPHYSIOLOGY** in the body of the message.

Newsgroups

Usenet:
> newsgroup: **sci.med.psychobiology**
> newsgroup: **sci.psychology**
> newsgroup: **alt.society.mental-health**
> newsgroup: **alt.psychology.personality**
> newsgroup: **alt.sexual.abuse.recovery**
> newsgroup: **alt.support.dissociation**

Mental Retardation

The Arc Home Page

Offers links to the Arc's government reports, publications, fact sheets, and listings of other Internet resources. Also included is specific information related to aging and mental retardation and fetal alcohol syndrome.
World Wide Web:
URL: http://www.thearc.org/

Resources on Mental Retardation

On-line articles, information about organizations, and Special Olympics. Good links to other resources and information including a list of mailing lists for a variety of concerns related to this topic.
World Wide Web:
URL: http://curry.edschool.virginia.edu/curry/dept/cise/ose/categories/mr.html

SERI: Special Education Resources on the Internet

Collections of Internet-accessible information and resources largely focused on education.
World Wide Web:
URL: http://www.hood.edu/seri/serihome.htm

Midwifery, Pregnancy, and Childbirth

Healthlinks: Breastfeeding

On-line articles and information, including initiating feeding, sore nipple management, and extensive links to other resources. A good place to start!
World Wide Web:
URL: http://healthlinks.washington.edu/conditions/breastfeeding.html

Midwifery, Pregnancy and Birth Related Information

Provides links to information about the history of midwifery, home births, nutrition and pregnancy, lactation, breastfeeding, and infant nutrition. There are also links to Midwifery Today's list of e-mail addresses. This is the best place to start looking for information on this topic.
World Wide Web:
URL: http://www.efn.org/~djz/birth/birthindex.html

Midwifery Today

Articles are available on-line.
World Wide Web:
URL: http://www.midwiferytoday.com/

Listservers

MIDWIFE
> To join, send mail to **midwife-request@fensende.com** with **subscribe MIDWIFE <first name> <last name>** in the body of the message.

FET-NET (Research in fetal and perinatal care)
> To join, send mail to **LISTSERV@HEARN.BITNET** with **SUB FET-NET <first name> <last name>** in the body of the message.

PRENAT-L
> To join, send mail to **LISTSERV@ALBNYDH2.BITNET** with **SUB PRENAT-L <first name> <last name>** in the body of the message.

Newsgroups

Usenet:
> newsgroup: **misc.kids.health**
> newsgroup: **misc.kids.pregnancy**
> newsgroup: **misc.kids.breastfeeding**
> newsgroup: **alt.support.breastfeeding**
> newsgroup: **alt.infertility**

Multiple Sclerosis

Multiple Sclerosis Society of Canada

Offers links to information about MS, a discussion area, and latest research.
World Wide Web:
URL: http://www.mssociety.ca/

National Multiple Sclerosis Society

A good selection of on-line information about MS, plus links to other organizations and resources.
World Wide Web:
URL: http://www.nmss.org

Newsgroup

Usenet:
   newsgroup: **alt.support.mult-sclerosis**

Neuroscience

Neurosciences on the Internet

This is the best site to browse a variety of topics such as brain injury and spinal cord injury.
World Wide Web:
URL: http://www.lm.com/~nab

Nutrition

Center for Food Safety and Nutrition

Provides links to information related to biotechnology, consumer advice, foodborne illness, food labeling, and FDA regulations.
World Wide Web:
URL: http://vm.cfsan.fda.gov/list.html

CSIRO Division of Human Nutrition

Offers links to an extensive variety of other resources and sites including consumer leaflets and research. A good site to browse.
World Wide Web:
URL: http://www.dhn.csiro.au

Food and Nutrition Information Center

Extensive links to publications, databases, full-text articles, FDA/USDA guidelines, and other Internet resources.
World Wide Web:
URL: http://www.nal.usda.gov/fnic

Godiva On-line

This is a Web site of Godiva chocolates. This is a fun (if not nutritious) site to visit. It offers links to the history of chocolate as well as recipes and on-line ordering!
World Wide Web:
URL: http://www.godiva.com

International Food Information Council

A Web site with the bulk of the links organized according to audience (parents, educators, etc.) related to subjects such as caffeine, food coloring, biotechnology, pregnancy, hyperactivity, and aspartame. Especially good consumer education.
World Wide Web:
URL: http://ificinfo.health.org/

The No Milk Page

This is a good staring point for information related to lactose intolerance, milk allergy, or casein intolerance.
World Wide Web:
URL: http://www.panix.com/~nomilk

Yahoo Nutrition Page

Offers links to a variety of nutrition sites and information.
World Wide Web:
URL: http://www.yahoo.com/Health/Nutrition

Newsgroups

Usenet:
  newsgroup: **sci.med.nutrition**
  newsgroup: **clari.biz.industry.food**
  newsgroup: **alt.support.diet**
  newsgroup: **alt.support.obesity**
  newsgroup: **alt.support.big-folks**
  newsgroup: **rec.food.veg**

Listservers

COMMNUTR-L (Community Nutrition)
  To join, send mail to **lisproc@cornell.edu** with **sub commnutr-l <first name> <last name>** in the body of the message.

Food-for-thought (mailing list)
> To join, send mail to **mailbase@mailbase.ac.uk** with **join food-for-thought <first name> <last name>** in the body of the message.

NUTEPI (Nutritional epidemiology)
> To join, send mail to **listserv@TUBVM.CS.TU-BERLIN.DE** with **sub NUTEPI <first name> <last name>** in the body of the message.

PHNUTR-L (Public health nutrition service providers)
> To join, send mail to **listproc@u.washington.edu** with **sub phnutr-l <first name> <last name>** in the body of the message.

Occupational Health

Association for Worksite Health Promotion

Information related to programs, conferences, publications, and the organization.
World Wide Web:
URL: http://www.awhp.org/

Canadian Centre for Occupational Health and Safety

Offers links to information and advice about occupational health and safety.
World Wide Web:
URL: http://www.ccohs.ca/

Computers and Health

Offers information on ergonomics, carpal tunnel syndrome, and VDT radiation.
Gopher:
URL: http://www.indiana.edu/~ucspubs/f026/

Injury Control Resource Information Network

Offers data, statistics, injury specific resources, research, publications, and announcements of upcoming conferences.
World Wide Web:
URL: http://www.injurycontrol.com/icrin/

Occupational Safety and Health

Extensive on-line articles and documents concerning a variety of occupational health risks and injuries. Also links to other resources.
World Wide Web:
URL: http://www.mic.ki.se/Safety.html

OSHWEB

This is the best place to begin searching this topic. Information provided related to chemical safety, emergency management, ergonomics, international organizations, hazard control, product safety, radiation, risk management, research institutes, and publications. Searchable.

World Wide Web:
URL: http://oshweb.me.tut.fi/index.html

Newsgroups

Usenet:
>   newsgroup: **comp.human.factors**
>   newsgroup: **comp.risks**
>   newsgroup: **sci.med.occupational**

Pharmacy

PharmWeb Home Page

Provides links to a PharmWeb Directory for finding people, PharmWeb Appointments, posting vacancies in pharmacy and related professions, pharmacy-related academic institutions and companies, government information, societies and groups and conferences and meetings. There is also a link to the newsgroups identified below.

World Wide Web:
URL: http://www.pharmweb.net

The "Virtual" Pharmacy Center

Includes information about and links to drug databases, drug research and development, drug interactions, reactions and infusion rates, new drugs, drug alerts, clinical pharmacology and toxicology, and links to associations and schools.

World Wide Web:
URL: http://www-sci.lib.uci.edu/HSG/Pharmacy.html

Newsgroups

Usenet:
>   newsgroup: **sci.med.pharmacy**
>   newsgroup: **sci.bio**
>   newsgroup: **sci.bio.microbiology**
>   newsgroup. **sci.bio.technology**

newsgroup: **sci.chem**
newsgroup: **sci.med**
newsgroup: **sci.polymers**

Listserver

PHARM

To join, send mail to **PHARM-REQUEST@DMU.ac.uk** with **subscribe PHARM <first name> <last name>** in the body of the message.

Polio

Polio Survivors Page: Polio and Post-Polio Resources

Links to articles, information packets, newsletters, and general resources related to polio and post-polio syndrome. A good place to start searching this topic.
World Wide Web:
URL: http://www.eskimo.com/~dempt/polio.html

Newsgroup

Usenet:
newsgroup: **alt.support.post-polio**

Rehabilitation

InContiNet

Provides general information for the public, full-text articles, abstracts and research designed for health care professionals, instrumentation information, and a listing of related professional and nonprofit organizations.
World Wide Web:
URL: http://www.incontinet.com/home.htm

MedWeb: Physical Medicine and Rehabilitation

A comprehensive directory of links to a variety of rehab-related topics such as assistive technology, sports medicine, stroke, other Internet resources related to brain injury, cognitive rehabilitation, neurology, spinal chord injury, orthopedics, and patient education.
World Wide Web:
URL: http://medwebplus.com/subject/Rehabilitation.html

Listservers

Incontilist (related to incontinence)
> To join, send mail to **incontilist-list@Incontinet**.com with **subscribe Incontilist <first name> <last name>** in the body of the message.

REHAB-RU
> To join, send mail to **listserv@ukcc.uky.edu** with **subscribe REHAB-RU <first name> <last name>** in the body of the message.

Repetitive Stress Injury

Computer-Related Repetitive Strain Injury (RSI)

Offers information on RSI, including links to other Web sites, including one with animations of stretches to do!
World Wide Web:
URL: http://www.engr.unl.edu/ee/eeshop/rsi.html

CTDNews

CTDNews current issue, prevention products, general information, and bulletin board.
World Wide Web:
URL: http://www.ctdnews.com/

ErgoWeb

Offers volumes of useful ergonomics information including instructional materials, standards and guidelines, news, and products.
World Wide Web:
URL: http://www.ergoweb.com/index.cfm

Occupational Safety and Health Administration (OSHA)

Provides statistics and data, upcoming conferences, standards, and technical information.
World Wide Web:
URL: http://www.osha.gov

Typing Injuries FAQS and Links

Has links to general information about typing injuries, ergonomics, publications, references, and keyboard alternatives. Another good beginning search site.
World Wide Web:
URL: http://www.tifaq.com/

Research

Agency for Health Care Research and Quality

This is comprehensive, searchable site including clinical information, evidence-based practice, clinical practice guidelines, information for consumers, funding opportunities, and data and surveys.
World Wide Web:
URL: http://www.ahcpr.gov/

National Institute of Nursing Research (NINR)

This site offers several documents including the National Nursing Research Agenda. Of greatest interest is the list of current program announcements and requests for applications. Guidelines for various grants and traineeships are also included.
World Wide Web:
URL: http://www.nih.gov/ninr/

National Institutes of Health: Scientific Resources

Provides research news, research training information, and listings of NIH research projects and sites.
World Wide Web:
URL: http://www.nih.gov/science

Newsgroup

Usenet:
    newsgroup: **sci.research**

Sexual Assault

Sexual Assault Information Page

Provides links to articles related to families, child sexual abuse, rape, sexual harassment, incest, domestic violence, prevention, and law.
World Wide Web:
URL: http://www.cs.utk.edu/~bartley/saInfoPage.html

Sexuality

Sexuality Information and Education Council of the U.S. (SIECUS)

SIECUS develops, collects, and disseminates information, promotes comprehensive education about sexuality, and advocates the right of individuals to make responsible sexual choices.. There is information on this site for adults, teens, policy makers, school health educators, and the media.
World Wide Web:
URL: http://www.siecus.org/

Newsgroup

Usenet:
    newsgroup: **alt.sex**

Sleep

Phantom Sleep Page

Incorporates the patient-directed site S.N.O.R.E., which provides links to information on sleep disorders including obstructive sleep disorder and the procedure laser-assisted uvulopalatoplasty. Also a sleep disorders FAQ, and information on sleep apnea and snoring for both the public and health care professionals.
World Wide Web:
URL: http://www.newtechpub.com/phantom/

SleepNet's Guide

Offers information about a variety of sleep disorders, sleep deprivation, sleep-related products, a listing of sleep-disorder centers and support groups, and extensive links to other sites.
World Wide Web:
URL: http://www.sleepnet.com

Sleep Medicine Home Page

Provides links to newsgroups, FAQs, articles and text files, and other Internet sites related to sleep. Many of these resources relate to children's sleep problems and SIDS.
World Wide Web:
URL: http://www.cloud9.net:80/~thorpy/

Newsgroup

Usenet:
     newsgroup: **alt.support.sleep-disorder**

Smoking

CDC's Tobacco Information and Prevention (TIPS) Sourcepage

Includes full-text articles, data, reports, and statistics related to tobacco use by a variety of specific populations. Also includes a publication list, a public information section on how to quit, other educational materials, and a search facility.
World Wide Web:
URL: http://www.cdc.gov/tobacco/index.htm

National Clearinghouse on Tobacco and Health

Provides full-text articles on a variety of tobacco-related issues for the public and health professional, including a youth series, and environmental tobacco smoke series. Also includes searchable databases of conferences, Web documents, and selected useful Web sites.
World Wide Web:
URL: http://www.ncth.ca/NCTHweb.nsf

Nursing Center for Tobacco Intervention

Features research abstracts, resource lists, and intervention guidelines.
World Wide Web:
URL: http://www.con.ohio-state.edu/tobacco

Newsgroups

Usenet:
> newsgroup: **clari.news.smoking**
> newsgroup: **alt.support.stop-smoking**
> newsgroup: **alt.support.non-smokers**
> newsgroup: **alt.support.non-smokers (moderated)**
> newsgroup: **alt.smokers**

Listservers

> List: address: **smoke-free@msstate.edu**
> Subscription address: **smoke-free-request@msstate.edu**
> List address: **on-listproc@msstate.edu**
> Subscription address: **on-listproc-request@msstate.edu**

Spirituality

IHP-NET: International Network for Interfaith Health   Practices

Provides links to information about the relationship between spirituality and health, the congregational nurse program, and other related sites.
World Wide Web:
URL: http://www.ihpnet.org/

Listserver

Interfaith Health Practices
> To join, send mail to **MAJORDOMO@interaccess.com** with **subscribe IHP-NET** in the body of the message.

Stress

Medline plus Health Information: Stress

This site offers information about coping with stress, children and stress, clinical trials, and links to other resources.
World Wide Web:
URL: http://www.nlm.nih.gov/medlineplus/stress.html

Stroke

American Stroke Association

This comprehensive site provides information for the public, professionals, and the media. There are links to publications and conferences.
World Wide Web:
URL: http://www.strokeassociation.org/

National Stroke Association

Provides on-line information for the public and professionals related to stroke prevention, screening, treatment, and research.
World Wide Web:
URL: http://www.stroke.org/

Listserver

STROKE-L
> To join, send mail to **listserv@ukcc.uky.edu** with **subscribe STROKE-L <first name> <last name>** in the body of the message.

Sudden Infant Death Syndrome

The Canadian Foundation for the Study of Infant Deaths

Provides information about SIDS, available resources, and other sites, including a French version.
World Wide Web:
URL: http://www.sidscanada.org/

National Sudden Infant Death Syndrome Resource Center

Provides information sheets and publications, annotated bibliographies, an information exchange newsletter, and reference and referral services.
World Wide Web:
URL: http://www.sidcenter.org

SIDS Network

Includes full-text articles about SIDS in English, Spanish, and German, information about support groups, research information, and links to other resources.
World Wide Web:
URL: http://sids-network.org

Wellness

Wellness Links

Offers links to a wide variety of wellness resources including holisticand alternative practices.
World Wide Web:
URL: http://www.wellmedia.com/links.html

WellnessWeb

Provides information related to a variety of wellness topics, including stress management, women's health, smoker's clinic, cancer center, and senior's center. Also links to a variety of disease/condition-specific mailing lists.
World Wide Web:
URL: http://wellweb.com

Listserver

Wellnesslist
To join, send mail to **majordomo@wellnessmart.com** with **subscribe Wellnesslist <first name> <last name>** in the body of the message.

Women's Health

Estronaut: A Forum for Women's Health

This site includes life-cycle information, "Ask a woman doctor," nutrition, risk assessment tools, and age-specific information.
World Wide Web:
URL: http://www.womenshealth.org/

Women's Health

Provides extensive information on women's health topics including breast self-exam, cryotherapy, menstrual cramps, Pap test, colposcopy, pelvic inflammatory disease, premenstrual syndrome, pregnancy, toxic shock syndrome, and urinary tract infection.
World Wide Web:
URL: http://www.mckinley.uiuc.edu/clinics/womens/womens.html

Listserver

HMATRIX-L (concerning on-line health resources)
To join, send mail to **listserv@ukanaix.cc.ukans.edu** with **subscibe HMATRIX-L <first name> <last name>** in the body of the message.

Online Journals

Australian Electronic Journal of Nursing Education (AEJNE)
World Wide Web:
URL: http://www.scu.edu.au/schools/nhcp/aejne

Bandolier: Evidence-based health care
World Wide Web:
URL: http://www.jr2.ox.ac.uk/Bandolier/

British Medical Journal
World Wide Web:
URL: http://www.bmj.com/

Disability International
World Wide Web:
URL: http://www.escape.ca/~dpi/DI.html

Harvard Public Health Review
World Wide Web:
URL: http://www.hsph.harvard.edu/review/

Health and Medical Informatics Digest
World Wide Web:
URL: http://144.92.205.41/hmid/2000/5_00hmid.htm

IMIA Newsletters
World Wide Web:
URL: http://www.imia.org/

Internet Journal of Advanced Nursing Practice
World Wide Web:
URL http://www.ispub.com/journals/ijanp.htm

Internet Journal of Health Promotion
World Wide Web:
URL: http://www.elecpress.monash.edu.au/IJHP/

Internurse: A resource for nurses and midwives
World Wide Web:
URL: http://www.internurse.com/

Journal of the American Medical Association
World Wide Web:
URL: http://jama.ama-assn.org/

The Lancet
World Wide Web:
URL: http://www.thelancet.com

Mental Health Net-Perspectives
World Wide Web:
URL: http://mentalhelp.net/perspectives/

New England Journal of Medicine
World Wide Web:
URL: http://www.nejm.org (by subscription only)

Nurseweek
World Wide Web:
URL: http://www.nurseweek.com

Nursing Standard Online
World Wide Web:
URL: http://www.nursing-standard.co.uk/

Nursing Trends and Issues
World Wide Web:
URL: http://www.nursingworld.org/readroom/nti/

On-line Journal of Issues in Nursing
World Wide Web:
URL: http://www.nursingworld.org/ojin/

On-line Journal of Nursing Informatics
World Wide Web:
URL: http://milkman.cac.psu.edu/~dxm12/OJNI.html

Rush Publications On-line

- RADC Newsletter, a newsletter of the Rush Alzheimer's Disease Center
- Connections, a newsletter of the Rush Arthritis and Orthopedics Institute
- Cancer Update, a newsletter of the Rush Cancer Institute
- HeartSource, information for the public from the Rush Heart Institute
- Rush Cardiac News, information for physicians from the Rush Heart Institute
- Rush Behavioral Health News, a newsletter of the Rush Institute for Mental Well-Being
- Puzzle Pieces, a newsletter of the Rush Neurobehavioral Center

World Wide Web:
URL http://www.rpslmc.edu/patients/publications/index.html

Western Journal of Nursing Research
World Wide Web:
URL: http://www.sagepub.co.uk/journals/details/j0044.html
(by subscription only)

Searchable Health-Related Literature Databases

Cinahl Direct

Cumulative Index to Nursing and Allied Health Literature. References over 900 journals. Output includes bibliographic data and abstracts. Paid membership required.
World Wide Web:
URL: http://www.cinahl.com/

Medline

National Library of Medicine offers PubMed and Internet Grateful Med, two free systems to search MEDLINE.
World Wide Web:
URL: http://www.nlm.nih.gov/databases/freemedl.html

Springhouse Reference Library

References over 100 nursing journals. Output includes bibliographic data and abstracts. No membership required.
World Wide Web:
URL: http://www.springnet.com/journals.htm

Glossary

Alias:	A special recipient name for a group of Internet addresses.
Anonymous FTP:	Computer site set to allow public retrieval of files using the login "anonymous."
Archie:	An information retrieval system for anonymous FTP sites.
Archive:	A set of one or more files that have been compressed to save space or speed up transmission over the Internet. Many of these files have names that end in .zip, .sit depending on the compression program used to create the file.
Backbone:	The basic communications link of a network.
Digest:	A collection of messages about a specific topic prepared by a mailing list moderator.
Domain name:	Name of a computer system that is registered with the Internet. Can be made up of subdomains such as geographic or organizational subdomains.
Dynamic rerouting:	Ability of a network to direct communications around a damaged connection to still reach the intended recipient.
E-mail:	Electronic mail.
Emoticons:	Icons for indicating emotions (see Chapter 2, Table 2.7).
FAQ:	Frequently asked question(s).
Forum:	Same as a Newsgroup.
FreeNet:	A computer network that brings together the resources of a community or campus and is available free of charge.
FTP:	File Transfer Protocol. A set of specifications that support Internet file transfer.

Gateway: Computer system that acts as a point of access that allows information to move back and forth between networks. Often used when the networks involved use different protocols.

Gopher: A way of organizing and categorizing certain types of information on the Internet.

Host: A synonym for any computer connected to the Internet, generally at a remote location.

Hypertext: Text that contains embedded links to other data.

Internet: The name for a group of worldwide computer-based information resources connected together.

Jughead: An information retrieval system for a specific Gopher site.

Listserv: Listserver, the most common computerized mailing list administration program.

Login ID: Unique identifying character string assigned to a user of a computer system.

Luddite: A person who believes that the progress brought by machines is dangerous to the public good.

Lurk or **lurking:**   Listening in on a mailing list or newsgroup discussion without replying.

Lynx: A text-based Web browser program.

Mailing list: A collection of Internet addresses that facilitates an electronic discussion group.

Mosaic: A Windows-based Web browser program that was the predecessor of most of the advanced browsers in use today.

Netscape: A Web browser program available for both Macintosh and PC (IBM compatible) computers.

Network: Two or more computers connected together so that information can move between them.

Newsgroup: A collecting site for messages about a specific theme.

Newsreaders: Programs used to access a newsgroup, such as rn, tn, nn, and tin.

Password: String of characters secretly chosen to verify that you are the valid user connected with a specific user ID.

PPP: Point-to-Point Protocol. A protocol that allows the use of someone else's Internet presence on a temporary basis. Internet service providers allow a user to connect to the Internet using this protocol.

SLIP: Serial Line Internet Protocol. A protocol that allows the use of someone else's Internet presence on a temporary basis. Internet service providers allow a user to connect to the Internet using this protocol.

TCP/IP: Transmission Control Protocol/Internet Protocol

Telnet: A program used to connect to a remote computer.

Terminal emula-   The process that allows your computer screen and keyboard
tion connection: to control a remote computer.

URL: Uniform Resource Locator. A standardized method for referencing an item on the World Wide Web, including a complete description and its location.

Usenet: User's Network, made up of all machines that receive network newsgroups.

User ID: User identification, synonymous with login ID.

Veronica: An information retrieval system for Gopher sites.

WAIS: Wide Area Information Servers. A way of categorizing and organizing certain types of information on the Internet.

Web browser: An information retrieval program for the World Wide Web that can interpret and display hypertext documents.

Index